QUEER AND
PLEASANT
DANGER:

Writing Out
My Life

LOUISE RAFKIN

CLEIS
PRESS

Also by Louise Rafkin
from Cleis Press

Different Daughters: A Book by Mothers of Lesbians
Different Mothers: Sons and Daughters of Lesbians Talk
  about Their Lives
Unholy Alliances: New Women's Fiction

Published in the United States by Cleis Press Inc., P.O. Box 8933, Pittsburgh, Pennsylvania 15221, and P.O. Box 14684, San Francisco, California 94114.

Printed in the United States on acid-free paper.
Cover design: Pete Ivey
Cover photograph: Marion Roth
Typesetting: CaliCo Graphics
Logo art: Juana Alicia

First Edition.
10 9 8 7 6 5 4 3 2 1

Grateful acknowledgment is made to the following for permission to reprint previously published material: Poem by Rumi from *Open Secret: Versions of Rumi*, translated by John Moyne and Coleman Barks. Threshold Books, RD 4, Box 600, Putney VT 05346. Used with permission. Quote from *Setsuko Migishi: A Retrospective*, exhibition catalogue published by the Asahi Shimbun and the National Museum of Women in the Arts, 1991. Used with permission.

Library of Congress Cataloging-in-Publication Data

Rafkin, Louise, 1958-
  Queer and pleasant danger : writing out my life / by Louise Rafkin.
    p. cm.
  ISBN: 0-939416-60-3 : $24.95. — ISBN: 0-939416-61-1 (pbk.) : $9.95
  1. Lesbians—Fiction.   2. Lesbians—Social life and customs.
I. Title
PS3568.A385Q4 1992
813'.54—dc20   92-2416
                                                                    CIP

ACKNOWLEDGMENTS

The author wishes to thank the editors of the following publications in whose pages some of the stories and essays in this volume originally appeared: *Coming Up!/ The San Francisco Bay Times, Poets and Writers, Sojourner, NYQ, The East Bay Express, Lesbian Love Stories* Vol. 1 and Vol. 2, *The San Francisco Bay Guardian, Nob Quarter, Word of Mouth, Nimrod: The Awards, Shankpainter #30, The Daily Californian,* and *Lovers: Stories by Women.*

Grateful appreciation to The Fine Arts Work Center in Provincetown and the Ludwig Vogelstein Foundation for generous support. Thanks to Bárbara Selfridge, Jacqueline Woodson, Sarah Randolph, Margaret Erhart and Melanie Braverman, for editorial advice. To Ann Wolfe for care and compassion. And to Pendekkar, for the flame.

But where there is danger, there grows also what saves.
— Friedrich Hölderlin, *Patmos*

Who sees inside from outside?
Who finds hundreds of mysteries
even where minds are deranged?

See through those eyes what is to be seen.
Who then is looking out from those eyes?
— Rumi

ABOUT THE AUTHOR

L ouise Rafkin lives with two teenaged desert tortoises in Mass-achusetts where she writes, teaches self-defense, and studies Poekoelan Tjiminde Tulen, an Indonesian martial art. She is the editor of three books from Cleis Press: *Different Daughters: A Book by Mothers of Lesbians* (1987), *Unholy Alliances: New Women's Fiction* (1988), and *Different Mothers: Sons and Daughters of Lesbians Talk about Their Lives* (1990). Her work has been cited for many honors, including recognition from the National Gay and Lesbian Press Association, a 1991 Lambda Literary Award for *Different Mothers*, a grant from the Ludwig Vogelstein Foundation, and two year-long residency fellowships at the Fine Arts Work Center in Province-town, MA.

CONTENTS

I. Stories about Worthwhile People: Fiction

SLUMBER PARTY

We lived in Rancho Del Mar, near the beach, but not everyone did. There were a whole mess of houses across the freeway, past the golf course, in what people called The Flats. The streets there were narrower and most were cracked and almost none had sidewalks. There were no patios for skateboarding or skating and the kids that lived over there mostly hung out at Al's Market. Some people over there lived in apartments, some even lived in these old hotels that had dry swimming pools, like craters, in their middles. I didn't go over there much but some kids that lived in The Flats went to our school, and some were even my friends. Cassy McDaniels was one.

Cassy McDaniels came to La Playa, my school, at the beginning of the sixth grade from I-don't-know-where. She had blonde hair that fell past her shoulders and sometimes she'd brush it over the back of her head and in front of her face so she'd look like Cousin It from "The Addams Family." We wore shorts under our dresses every day, so that when we hung from the monkey bars or played dodge ball no one could see our panties. Cassy never wore shorts and you could always see under her dress, but she didn't notice or else didn't care. I had dreams about going to school and forgetting to put on shorts. I could never understand how Cassy made it through recess. But I always wanted to play with her.

By Christmas she was popular. She told us all about Slam Books. They had them at her old school. You would write your name in the front of them next to a number and then on every page there would be a question like, Who Do You Like? Or, Who is the Best Kisser? Or, What Teacher Don't You Like? So you'd fill out the questions and pass it around, and then everyone would try to steal it and you'd slam it shut. None of us had ever kissed anyone so some of the questions we left blank. Lila Medici wrote on that one "None of your bee's wax!" but we knew she hadn't kissed

11

anyone either. Cassy wrote the name of some boy from her other school, and then she put three stars next to it because she said he was a real good kisser. I wondered what made someone really good.

It was hard to convince my mom to let me go to Cassy's slumber party. She didn't know the family. "And are Mr. and Mrs. McDaniels going to be there?" For about a week she said "We'll see" and "I'll discuss it with your father," and then Mrs. Larson called to invite her and Dad to a cocktail party and she said yes. Then it was easier for me to go than for them to find a baby sitter, plus my older brother had a basketball game and she couldn't just dump me with him.

But I didn't really want to go. At slumber parties you don't get much sleep and I liked to sleep. If I didn't get enough sleep I'd wake up with a stomach ache. Mostly I worried about not getting to sleep, but if you went to sleep early the others were likely to put your hand in a cup of warm water. And then you'd wet the bed. Sometimes I liked to sleep over at someone's house, or better, have someone over mine. But even though I went to slumber parties I was always scared.

What would you be asked to do? What would happen when they started to play truth or dare? What if boys came over and wanted to play spin the bottle? What if Cassy McDaniels started to strip — where would you look?

When we played truth or dare, I took dare. Luckily all I had to do was knock on Mrs. McDaniels bedroom door. She was in there with her boyfriend, but the television was turned so loud she didn't hear, or maybe she ignored me. It was late and we had eaten a ton of caramel corn and then had started to make chocolate chip cookies, but Cassy decided we should just eat the dough raw. After a while my stomach hurt. I lay flat on my back under my red and black flowered sleeping bag, hoping that perhaps the others would think I was asleep. Cassy was about to strip.

She turned the lights off, all except the kitchen light which spilled into the living room. She put some slow music on the hi-fi, something of her mother's, and hid herself in the living-room drapes. She folded into them like a caterpillar in a cocoon.

All of us ten girls were quiet. Everyone was in sleeping bags and the floor looked like some sort of funny quilt. Most of the others were sitting up, but I just peeked over the top of my bag.

The music started to swell and Cassy rolled herself out from the drapes. Her black pedal pushers were tight on her already-rounded hips, and her dotted blouse was tied at her waist. She pushed her hair up and off her face like some sort of movie star. Her shirt hiked up, and I could see a crescent of a shining white bra. Puckering her lips, she kissed at the air. Lila screamed, and then everyone else did, too. Then the others all tumbled to a heap at Cassy's feet, giggling and laughing. Helen turned the stereo up.

At every overnight Cassy stripped. At Rachel Whitmore's party she took some of her clothes off. At the age of eleven she already had her period and already had breasts and most of the rest of us didn't have either. Sometimes she just danced and moved around, twisting from side to side like a snake. Now she started to bob and dip to the music, rubbing her hands along her thighs and then wrapping her arms around herself so that from the back it looked like someone was hugging and feeling her. The first song ended, and she had only undone the top three buttons of her blouse. "More! More!" said Lila, and then everyone else said it, too. Cassy looked towards the back bedroom but there was just a faint line of TV blue glowing from under her mother's door.

The next song was faster. Cassy swung her hips and flipped her hair over onto her chest. Then she untied and peeled away her blouse. Her white bra shone in the half light of the living room, and we all hushed. Most of us still wore undershirts. Cassy flipped her hair back and laughed; then we did, too. I was sitting with the other girls now. I wore two-piece striped pajamas, but some of the others, like Lila, had on babydolls. Cassy was standing with her shirt off. At Rachel's house she had stopped after taking her shirt off; it looked like she was going to go further.

I stared at her bra. Lumps of creamy flesh tucked into pointy cups almost like those cones you put in those plastic holders for drinking. I was warm. I tried to get into the middle of the others, to laugh and giggle, but the strange feeling in my stomach just got worse.

Cassy had turned around and unzipped her pedal pushers. She started to push them down over her hips. It looked like a banana losing its skin. The pants were tight and they got stuck on her thighs; she had to bend over to pull them down. The smile across the back of her white Carter's underwear made me gasp and I coughed to cover it up. Angela Ellis sat up and slapped Cassy's bottom when she was doubled over. "Bull's eye!" she said. Everyone laughed. Cassy kicked off her pants and turned around to face us. She tried to pretend she was mad at Angela, but when she turned and saw everyone smiling she smiled too, this long wide smile, slow-like. Her bikini underwear fell short of the line where her bathing suit stopped, so a pale stripe, about the color of a tan Crayola crayon, circled her waist.

"Show us your boobies!" Melinda said, and Cassy slid her bra down her tanned arms. I could hardly breathe. White triangles of flesh spotted with pink moons sat on her chest like targets and I couldn't take my eyes from them. The other girls started to horse around a little; I sat behind them and watched. Cassy touched the very tips of her breasts and started to moan.

"This is what they do down at the Cat 'N' Mouse," she said. The Cat 'N' Mouse was a bar near her house. "I know cause I went there with my mom."

I'd walked past it before. The sign in front showed a cat chasing a mouse down a hole. The cat had long whiskers that flashed on and off.

I backed away from the other girls, all the way to the fireplace, scraping my legs against some ceramic logs stacked against the bricks. Cassy was standing half naked in front of everybody, talking about the Cat 'N' Mouse. "Well, they don't take everything off," she admitted. "But almost."

Melinda had moved up close to where Cassy was standing and she reached up and grabbed at Cassy's underpants, pulling them down past Cassy's knees. Cassy screamed and then everyone did, too. I swallowed, trying to keep the air inside of me from coming out and making a noise. I didn't want anyone to look at me. I wanted to be invisible. In the light from the kitchen I could see a tiny triangle of dark hair like a small shadow between Cassy's legs.

Cassy tried to move but her panties were caught around her ankles and she toppled into everyone. There was a big tangle. I wanted to jump into the mess and touch her too, but I also wanted her to put her clothes back on. I didn't know what I wanted.

"What's the matter with you?" Cassy said. She was lying on her stomach over Lila's knees, her hair all messy across her face. She looked right at me and I looked away. Someone pinched her bottom, and she turned over and away from me. They were all laughing again.

I felt frozen to the fireplace and unable to move. My stomach was queasy and itchy. While they were still wrestling with each other I went to the bathroom. The crotch of my pajama bottoms was damp. I touched myself and it was a little slimy. I grabbed a towel and started to rub myself dry.

THE LIFE CYCLE OF THE WOOLLY APHID

1. Falling Aphids

Marsha is on a ladder propped next to the plum tree, her hands inside two plastic vegetable bags. Despite the warmth of the afternoon, she's wearing a black stocking cap and an old wool scarf wrapped around her face, and all I can see are her eyes, dark and determined. Even in this get-up she is beautiful. And in spite of the plastic mittens, Marsha deftly wields her weapon: a garden hose with an attached sprayer. A mist of green insecticide hisses onto sagging leaves, and the sickly smell of the poison mingles with the smoggy eighty-degree sunshine.

"Take that." I hear her muffled war cry.

"You tell 'em," our friend Richard calls from the vegetable patch.

"Don't forget the undersides," I add from across the yard.

Marsha is at war with the aphids. Richard is weeding. I'm snipping roses. Although it's early October, tomatoes are still ripening and there are new buds on both yellow rose bushes. Here in L.A. things bloom at strange times. In the spring, of course, but often year round as if to show they can adapt. Like Marsha and I, both Midwestern girls who have lived here fifteen years and have only recently stopped shopping for winter clothes. Some years it is already Thanksgiving before I realize the summer is over. My mother, still in Kansas, can't believe we have roses year round. She claims it's because of the smog and the nuclear power plants and the earthquakes. "It's just not natural," she says, which is also what she says about Marsha and me.

Today is the first day Marsha has tried to slay the aphids with poison. Over the past few years we've fought these aphids fairly, organically, on their own terms. We've rubbed the leaves of our varied and numerous trees and shrubs with garlic and washed them carefully with bleach. We've even painted several tree trunks with a concoction of Chinese herbs that Richard whipped up in his blender. Last spring we sent away to West Virginia for small bags stuffed with starving ladybugs that were delivered by UPS somehow still alive. These critters were supposed to chow down on the aphids, grow fat and lazy and then buzz harmlessly from flower to flower. Ladybug paradise, aphid hell. But as soon as we freed those gals they took flight, *en masse*, to our neighbor's back yard. Presumably their aphids were tastier.

We have a brightly-colored illustrated chart taped to the refrigerator: "The Life Cycle of the Woolly Aphid." They hand these out at the nursery, as inspiration. But it's depressing. These guys are invincible, their procreative abilities amazing. Actually they're not guys at all: Almost all aphids are female, and strangely enough, they reproduce by parthenogenesis. Girls beget girls.

"That should do it," Marsha says, descending the ladder.

"Forever the optimist," Richard says and catches my eye through the branches of the rosebush. Shirtless now, he has abandoned the weeding and is lying on the lawn next to the roses.

Marsha's painter's pants are spotted with green insect goo. She pulls off the stocking cap and her hair, a thick red-brown river, catches the sun as it falls onto her shoulders.

"I'm going to get these suckers if it's the last thing I do," Marsha says.

"And their children, and their children's children," Richard says.

"I have my doubts," I say.

"You always have doubts," Richard adds, but not loud enough for Marsha to hear.

I resume my clipping.

Marsha and I moved here in the early seventies, from Iowa and Kansas, respectively. We met working at Wonder Woman Painters, a women's collective. For some years we flirted, while dating others, and finally nine years ago found ourselves both semi-single — she was technically still living with Georgia — at the same New Year's Eve party. Eventually we left house painting for what we thought was the real world. She to social work, I to middle management in a computer firm. Gradually, we left our political groups and took subscriptions to the *Nation* and *Mother Jones*. We care as much as we ever did about changing the world, but our passion has slowly subsided, both for politics and each other. But we are comfortable, and I would say most times, happy. We're an inspiration to many of our friends, both straight and gay, most of whom have been through a half dozen partners in the nine years we've been together.

We're settled. We've bought this house, and despite the armies of aphids, we have a wonderful garden: citrus trees, honeysuckle vines, strawberries, even an avocado that produces tiny, sweet fruits each summer, one of which I send to my mother. I'm sure it goes to waste (she would never eat such a thing), but since there are no longer report cards to bring home and no grandchildren, it seems right that I send this small offering instead. I sent along a recipe for guacamole, but she said her neighbor once made tacos (which she pronounced "take-os") and they made my father sick. They've had meat, potatoes and vegetables, boiled, every night for the last forty-five years. It frightens me. They say you can end up like your parents without even realizing.

"Can we take this down now?" Marsha is pointing to a Chinese lantern hanging from the apple tree. "It's certifiably de-bugged."

Looking up from the pink rosebush, I nod. The lantern is a remnant from Marsha's thirty-ninth birthday party last week. It was a theme party, Hawaiian luau, and we all wore mumus and tacky tourist shirts and some, like Richard, bathing suits. A plastic lei hangs off the rhododendron. Marsha slips it over her head.

"I hope you got lei-ed on your birthday," says Richard, with a strong camp inflection.

"That's none of your business, Mr. Busybody," Marsha says and mimes a hula. I shoot Richard a nasty look. We're each other's romantic confidant; he knows this is a touchy subject. Marsha and I haven't had sex in over a year. And for the four years before that it was infrequent — that's a generous assessment. Saturday night, a rare Sunday morning. Both of our jobs take a lot out of us. We've been together so long. I could make excuses forever. There is no passion. But also no question that I love her.

I've talked with other people about this. Most who have been in long-term relationships (which these days qualifies at about three years) say there are cycles. First you're hot, then you're not, then you are again but "differently." We've been through this cycle a few times, but right now we're stuck. Our current phase is referred to in self-help circles as "bed death" — a term that sent Richard into convulsions. He's gay and swears sex is easy; it's relationships that are hard. Marsha disappears into the garage. I send Richard the evil eye.

"Thanks," I say.

"Stay put," he says quietly. "Rent porn, buy some sex toys. You two are the only ones I know who actually get along. Honey, you two can't break up. Someone has got to stay together."

"There's always Irene and Peter."

"Swell," Richard says, rolling his eyes.

Irene and Peter are our only friends who have been together longer than we have, ten years. Irene has admitted that there's been long periods of time when they *go without*. But all of us in the *know* know that Peter never goes without. A university professor, he usually has something on with one of his students.

But it's not like I've been Miss Celibacy either. The thirties are supposed to be the height of a woman's sexuality and I'm loathe to miss out on this once-in-a-lifetime experience. I've had a couple brief affairs over the last few years, nothing Marsha knows about concretely. Insignificant flings with women from the gym and last winter a spate of weekly "lunch" dates with the software specialist at work. She married one of the V.P.s last June, a man, and that put an end to it. Actually she suggested we might see each other occasionally, but I'm not stupid; I'd be the one to lose my job.

I assume Marsha's done the inevitable elsewhere as well. She has these sudden interests in trendy activities like African drumming or kung fu, which are usually accompanied by a "special friendship." I ignore these, and usually the new friend fades out after a few months along with the interest in whatever it was. Marsha and I really should break up, move out, get angry, get over it, and be friends. But neither of us wants to upset the nest. When the subject comes up, rarely, both of us panic and run into each other's arms. It's the climate. Everyone is supposed to couple and procreate. All of our single friends want desperately not to be. They swear dating is no fun, and stories I've heard confirm all reports. But what about the long haul?

The winter sun is weakening and Richard has shirted up.

"I'll tell you a secret," he says, his hands kneading my shoulders.

"What kind of secret do *you* know?"

"This is my secret, Abigail, my love: Passion is overrated." He has stopped the massage, dramatically, à la Richard.

"With what you get in the sex department, that's a bit like Rockefeller saying money won't buy happiness."

"I know of which I speak," he says, steps back and bows formally. "I have to run. Early dinner date." It's time for me to roll my eyes. "Please tell your wife good-bye," he says and disappears around the side of the house. Momentarily, I hear the buzz of his motorscooter.

"I'm starting dinner," Marsha calls from the back of the house. "I'm starving."

"Me, too," I say, but I feel slightly nauseous. From the insectiside, I think. Carefully, I bag the rose clippings and stack the thorny green bags against the garage.

The sprayer is washed and drying on the patio table. Marsha has stripped off her dirty clothes in the garage, and already the washer is churning. She's the only housemate I've ever gotten along with. She's as particular as I am, and in the same ways. The top is always on the toothpaste, the dishes are done before bedtime, and we both hate cat hair on the sofa. On the other hand, it's acceptable to leave clothes in the bathroom, and hair in the sink is no big deal. Richard says these things are not to be underrated, that compatibility is half the struggle. My therapist says I have to pee or get off the pot. She has urged me to break through or break up.

I'm thirty-seven and half my life is over. I get up earlier now. There is less time left.

Inside, I find Marsha on the phone with her mother.

"Abigail's going back east for a conference," she reports and then she pauses. "No, Mom. I really don't mind it. Being alone is nice once in a while."

I put the roses into a vase and place them on the round oak table in the kitchen. The vase was a gift from Marsha's mother for our last anniversary. It's one of those slim glass kind with marbles in the bottom. Marsha's mother refers to me as Marsha's "life partner," a term she picked up at a Parents of Gays support group meeting, and one that now makes me a little uncomfortable sometimes. Marsha complains about her mom. She calls two or three times a week just to "check in" with us "girls," and she does her share of prying. But I'd gladly swap parents. Once driving east we stopped in at my folks' house in Wichita. My dad took Marsha golfing, and being the jock that she is, she took to it like a pro. He was impressed with her natural ability.

"I'd groom you for the LPGA," he told her, "but those girls are a bunch of lezzies." My mother instructed me early on not to tell him about "it" because "it" would give him a heart attack. "Then where would I be?" she asked, always available to play the martyr. Ollie North is my father's hero. He's a retired Army engineer, and he *subscribes* to *USA Today*. He's a classic. Even after nine years, he's still clueless about Marsha and me.

"I hear them aphids dying as we speak," Marsha says hanging up the wall phone. "Crashing to the dirt by the thousands. Tomorrow they'll be piled up like snowdrifts. We'll have to get out there with shovels; the kids will be jumping into the piles as if they were fallen leaves." She washes lettuce from the garden. The pasta water is boiling.

"What time do you go tomorrow?" she asks.

"The van picks me up at six."

I put vermicelli in the pot, adding more and more because I'm never sure how much is enough. There is a huge clump at the bottom; it's going to come out in a glob, like one of those clusters of electrical wires on a homemade bomb.

"I'll miss you, Boo-boo," she says.

I look up. "Me, too, Madame Kumquat."

Marsha turns back to the sink. I see the flex in her arm muscles, an arch that slides forward and back in time with the washing movements of her hands.

After dinner, I finish packing my small bag for five days in a Vermont lodge: sweatshirts, jeans, one reasonably-dressy gray skirt. Ten years ago none of us would have been caught dead in a skirt. Now it's the rare lesbian who doesn't have some power clothes hanging in her closet next to her proverbial leather jacket. Luckily, I remember to take my jacket; I've almost forgotten that elsewhere there are still seasons, as if the City of Angels dictated the country's weather as well as its celluloid culture.

Marsha is propped up in bed reading one of those popular co-dependency books. There are three or four of these piled up on her side of the bed. She comes home every Thursday with a new one, after her therapy. She's convinced we're both co-dependent, but from what I understand, unless you're a total egomaniac it's hard not to be. I encourage her reading and have asked her to notify me immediately if she discovers easy answers.

On my side of the bed are a stack of *Nations* dating back two months, a few library books, biographies mostly, and a dog-eared copy of one of those popular vampire books. These unfulfilled walking dead actually appeal to me. This may be a bad sign.

Marsha puts down her book. "News about Maya, through Francis."

"She's not going through with it?"

"Full speed straight ahead," she says, grimacing. "So to speak."

Maya is our friend who, in one of life's great depressions (after a major break-up, I must add), made a pilgrimage to Israel to discover her Jewish roots. She connected with some sort of ultra-rightist sect. The women still shave their heads when they marry so they're not attractive to anyone but their husbands. Maya is now in an arranged engagement to a man she hardly knows. In the seventies, Maya was one of our most foot-loose and fancy-free sisters. She was convinced all men were mutants, lacking a properly crossed chromosome, and she was at the helm of half our marches, proudly waving the banner of the hour.

"She wrote that she is happy, that she is very — quote — *serene*, and that everything in her day-to-day life is dictated down to the littlest thing," Marsha reports. "That for the first time in her life she doesn't have to think about what to do, how to do it, or why."

"Great," I say. "Sounds like boot camp."

"Shall we send a vibrator for the wedding gift?"

"She'll probably need it," I say, without humor. My vibrator is plugged in, though hidden under the bed. I masturbate often, but usually when Marsha's not home. Sometimes when she's in the shower.

"I still can't believe it," Marsha says. "Of all people."

Naked I slide into bed. It's after midnight. I can picture Maya with her head shaved. She wore her hair that way for years actually, in the early seventies.

"Spoon or fork," Marsha asks.

"Spoon," I say. She curls against my back.

"Tim again," I say when the alarm fizzles.

"Again?" Marsha mumbles. "I'm sick of that boy in our bed."

I can't help it. I've been dreaming about my high school boyfriend for years now. Usually when I'm in a hard place, upset or stressed, he comes floating in, makes perfect love to me, deposits me into a fairy-tale house with a white picket fence. I wake up thinking, where is he? Shouldn't I marry him? Wouldn't it be easier? But I visited him a couple years ago when I was home. Five kids, a tract home with two mortgages, a wife who works evenings to help with the bills.

Still, a dream has its own agenda.

2. Falling Leaves

In Vermont, the hills are all shades of red and yellow and I'm once again experiencing autumn. There are leaves piled everywhere; they are bunched along the highway, splayed across fences, wedged into every crevice of every building. Air-borne varieties spin in the breeze like tiny red and gold sky divers.

But aside from the scenery, and certain company, the conference has been a bust. We are learning about motivation and competition and other swell four syllable concepts which we are to instill in those we lord over forty hours a week in our respective cities on our respective coasts and several points in between. Tomorrow we go home, supposedly inspired and renewed. Hardly. *But.*

I have never had an affair on a work trip. But here I am, the night before I will return to Marsha, sitting in a lodge in Vermont in front of a half-inspired fire with my hormones blazing. I've been flirting all week, heavily. I feel lust and something else, too, like I am testing some unknown waters, like I've abandoned myself to fate. Three overstuffed sofas frame the room and ring the fire. Each of us — Stan and Sally and myself — claim a sofa to ourselves.

"Sex can be as complicated as love, but it's a different kind of complication." Stan says this half seriously and Sally and I laugh at him. Actually what he says is all too true but it's good that the two of us laugh together because the seams of this threesome are pulling tight.

Stan sits on the center sofa, up straight with his hands in his lap like a schoolboy awaiting instructions. He lives on a ranch near Pierre, South Dakota, though the only animals on the place are the fish in his wife's aquarium. He's actually quite handsome, ruddy and squared-off like a Ralph Lauren model without the horse.

Sally is reclined, her head against the rounded end of her couch. One of her legs, cased in well-worn Levi's, is looped over the back of the couch. An arm is crooked behind her head. Dark hair, a heart-shaped face, deep blue eyes, a spray of freckles. She sighs and shifts onto her side. I want to bury my head in the worn crotch of her jeans, feel the hard metal buttons against my cheek. It's been almost a year since my last fling and this woman has set me aflame as quickly as if I were a turning leaf.

But though I may be a leaf, I am no crumb. I have given great thought to Marsha. Just outside the lounge, in the hall, is a pay phone. I've called several times over the last few days, never reaching her in person. "Aphid Control headquarters," reported the answering machine the first time I called. "Death and destruction and other dirty deeds done here. Leave a message."

I left a threat from the leader of the Aphid Nation: "Marsha Milton, there's a price on your head."

The next time I called — mid-morning here, early morning there — still no answer, but a fresh message, a gospel version of "We Shall Overcome" in the background, Marsha's voice in the foreground, in her best Girl Scout voice, "A warning to all aphids: We have God on our side." I hung up before the tone. I liked the message, but wondered where she was.

"Who's going to do what with who?" Stan asks, breaking into my thoughts.

"With whom," Sally corrects. She's in communications at the Philadelphia branch.

"Give me a break," Stan says. "I'm a small town boy from the Midwest."

"Sure," Sally says. "One who dreams of being tied up by two middle-management women." She looks over at me. "How are your knots?"

From the first day, I read Sally wrong: straight hair, jeans, crew neck sweater, no make-up. Anybody except my dad would have come to the same conclusion. At breakfast the first morning, we sat together, talked. This and that, one thing, then the next. I mentioned my house partner, no gender of course, and our fight against the aphids. She said she lived by herself, unless you counted the ants in her kitchen. "Which," she quipped, "are countless."

At lunch we talked about where we've traveled (she'd been to India — stayed at an ashram), about how down deep we really hated our jobs, about not wanting babies.

"My partner sort of wants one," I said, finally making that awkward first step from the closet. "Only she'd want me to have it." This baby thing has come up recently with Marsha, semi-seriously. All of our friends seem to be talking about it or making them. Time was when being gay kept this decision at arm's length; now that arm's connected to a turkey baster.

Sally didn't flutter a lash at the gender slip. "I'm lucky. The one I'm seeing already has two kids." I assumed "the one" was a woman. At dinner that night she told me otherwise.

"Ted — that guy I'm seeing? — is married," she said. "That's why I got promoted. I'm always at work. I only see him Sunday afternoons. So what else do I have to do but work? His wife thinks he plays squash. But he gets a good workout with me." She lifted her eyebrows, held them there for effect. Then winked. This heavy flirting has been fueled from both sides.

Once or twice I caught myself wondering what it would be like to leave L.A., move to Philadelphia, and take annual vacations in Vermont during leaf season. Sally is funny and charming and warm and has a great ass, and, as I make this list, I realize these are all qualities that first attracted me to Marsha.

Mid-week, Sally pulled Stan into her net. We're the only three, of fifty, that don't dress in suits and ties or the female equivalent. Today we skipped the afternoon class: "Getting What You Need from Your Work Environment." "Fat chance," Sally said after reading the course description. Then she told the company coordinators there had been a sudden death in her family and she needed to send a telegram, and that we, Stan and I, had to go with her for emotional support. We drove to the tavern up the road.

We played pool and had a few beers. Sally flirted with us both. Stan was after Sally but let me know he wasn't discriminating.

"I had an affair with a lesbian last year," he told me when Sally was at the bar. "She'd give me a good reference." He coyly dipped his head. A stray curl fell onto his forehead.

"So did I," I replied. "And so would she."

Later Sally and I were in the bathroom together. She stood at the mirror and pulled her thick hair flat behind her ears. "See? I'd look cute as a lesbian, huh?" She pinched my waist before flipping the buttons on her jeans closed, one handed. Marsha does that, but try as I may, I need two.

Now, here in the drawing room, the fire has warmed the room to sauna level. Stan has unbuttoned the top two buttons of his plaid shirt. Sally's face is flushed.

"I've never really considered sleeping with a woman before," Sally says. "I should have done it when I was in college. You know. Group sex, lesbian sex. Maybe if I'd grown up in the sixties I would have."

"What's wrong with now?" I say lightly. "We've got some rights, gay parades, our own newspapers, weekly features on Oprah and Phil. In certain circles it's almost trendy." But as I say this I know what Sally is really pointing out: Her life is neatly ordered and she's not going to mess it up. Work. Sunday afternoon sex. Similar to Maya marooned over there in the Israeli desert. And me, too. Why would I want to mess up my tidy life?

"Who's got the ropes?" I say, because Cowboy Stan is sitting there grinning. This is truly what he wants, I realize, only he's too afraid to say. Sally knows it too.

"What would your wife say if she knew you wanted to be tied up?" Sally asks.

"I think she'd want to watch."

Sally harrumps and turns onto her back. The wife is a problem for her. She was flirting with him just fine, until today when he started talking about Adeline: her job as a law lecturer, her marathon running. This afternoon when Stan claimed he truly loved his wife, Sally called him scum. I know it's because of this Ted, who also loves his wife and isn't going to leave her.

"So kiss me," Sally says now to Stan. "Let's get cracking. Show me that you want it."

"Really?" Stan sounds like a teenager, like he should stamp his feet and say "hot damn." Sally stretches out long on the couch, her hands folded onto her chest. She reminds me of those vampires, lying in wait for nightfall. Stan squares his shoulders and crosses to her couch.

"You mind?" he says to me.

"Fine by me," I say, always the gracious loser. I'm thinking that Richard is going to enjoy this story, even though it's questionable whether I am. We keep expecting straight people to have this relationship stuff figured out. They have a lot more to go on: scripts to follow.

Stan sets himself on the edge of the sofa and leans in towards Sally. Their lips tap once or twice before he slips his tongue in. I'm watching, but wondering about Marsha. Is she having an affair this week? Will we stay together? I'd like to call her, but if she's not there I would hang up.

Meanwhile Stan and Sally are slurping and I realize that what with all the build up, I'm wet. I tug at the seam of my jeans, close my eyes, and put both hands in my pockets.

There's a folded piece of paper in my right pocket. A small square of light blue.

It's a post-it note, folded crosswise. As I unfold it I see that there are tiny pictures of stick-figure bugs drawn on it. Two of the bugs are holding up flags. "WE SURRENDER," is written next to a particularly fat bug. "Death to all Aphids," it says at the bottom next to a skull and crossbones. The bugs are long-limbed; one wears basketball shoes and one is obviously bug-eyed. I'm thinking of Marsha, hunched over, drawing these funny bugs and then slipping them secretly into my pocket. But turning over the note, I realize it's my errand list from last week: post office, bank, tampons. Marsha's doodlings just happen to be on the other side.

I look up because Sally has started laughing. Stan is upright with his arms out in that don't-ask-me position. "What? What did I do wrong?" He looks to me, "You saw, I hardly did anything!"

"Maybe that's the problem," I say.

"I can't kiss with someone watching," Sally says, and now she's sitting up. "I haven't done that since fifth grade, when I played spin the bottle."

"Don't stop on my account," I say. "I was just leaving."

But Sally gets up first, flips back that hair, and crosses to my sofa. My cool is draining out the soles of my feet. A part of me — possibly the warm part between my legs — still wants to grab her and throw her on the couch next to me. The fire falls, loud in the silence.

"What's going on here?" Stan says. "What's the game plan?"

Sally sits down next to me, lightly. She leans in and I think she's going to kiss me, but instead she brushes the hair back from my ear.

"It's nothing personal," she whispers. "Don't take it personally, because I really like you." She strokes my thigh, up and back, and then stands.

"I'm hitting the sheets," she announces. "You two make the best of this fine evening." She turns, and I'm ashamed to say both Stan and I are staring at her ass. Things are complicated in this modern world.

"You're still scum," she says over her shoulder to Stan. "And you," she looks at me, "whip him good."

After she's gone the room feels colder to me. The electricity has drained, spun out the fogged-up windows into the cold New England air. Stan moves to my sofa.

"And so," he says, undaunted, and he smiles wide.

I shake my head no, slowly. He doesn't realize, but I still consider him my rival.

The moisture on the inside of the windows catches the feeble light from the fire, glittering like tiny stars against the black outside.

Suddenly I turn and slip my hand through Stan's arm, wrapping my leg over his, twining our limbs. This is what Marsha calls fork: cuddling or sleeping with limbs tangled, like forks in a messy silverware drawer. The crumpled post-it note rests on the couch next to me.

"Tell me about your marriage," I say quickly, before he follows a misguided notion. "Tell me how you love your wife."

"It's complicated," he says, and his eyebrows crinkle. He's confused.

Stan's body feels foreign, but warm and somehow comforting. I wonder how we can make anything last, through the long years of our lives. I wonder about the people we betray, ourselves and the others.

"Nicknames, you have nicknames?"

"Yes," he says. "Woozle Pie. Beetle Butt."

"Yes," I say clearly, as if he has confirmed a scientific hypothesis.

Then I think about my yellow roses, still in bloom, while outside the trees are nearly naked.

OBITS AND WEDDINGS

There's no good ones today," I say to Alan.

The New York Times is open on the floor in front of me. Photos of smiling couples peer up, boys on the left, girls on the right, both sets of mouths pulled into taut grins buoyed by an almost perceptible net of anxiety. I scan the page. Dr. and Mrs. So-and-So. Stanford Something-the-Third and Emily Blah-Blah-Blah. Checkerboarded on the opposite page, single frames of women, their hair swept back into dramatic waves, each with a strand of pearls resting on her neck. They are a bit older than I, at nineteen, and don't look unlike me, but their names are different: Amy, Kathleen, Alexandra, Daphne.

My name is Elliot Reeves. Yes, a girl named Elliot.

"Not even one black," I say to Alan. Alan — Professor Reizenfeld — is retired, an ex-colleague of my father. He dresses like an old professor, brown corduroy trousers and cardigan. He's perched in the winged-back chair reading the obits. He looks up. His bifocals make his eyes look birdlike, wide and oddly skewed.

"There's an Asian," I say.

I read aloud the accompanying blurb. July wedding for Mariana Ng; she's the thirty-four-year-old daughter of a Taiwanese shipping family, she's been educated abroad, and she's marrying an American V.P. who works in international banking. His dad's a chairman, his mother's a So-and-So. Maybe she's not supposed to be hitching up with a foreigner. But then possibly her parents think they've hit the jackpot. I can't tell on this one.

Other than this, there are no real scandals. Everyone else seems to be marrying within their own race and class. They're all graduates.

Last week this guy whose dad is some big muckety muck at Yale married this woman he met in a diner. They referred to her in the *Times* as working in the food service industry. Alan knows the guy's father and said the marriage is killing him. These are the stories I love.

"No one very interesting died," Alan says. "Including me."

"Not this week," I say, folding the paper and stacking it next to the fireplace.

The microwave dings off; it's time for Sunday dinner. Alan shifts himself out of the winged-back chair, creeping his skinny butt to the edge before launching himself upwards, shakily, one frail hand gripping the edge of the chair like a prehistoric bird. He coughs.

I cross the room in front of him, and he hardly notices even though I have great tits. I'm topless; it's part of the deal. Two years ago, when I started cooking for Alan, he was still drinking. One night he offered me money and asked me to take my shirt off, nothing else. Twenty-five dollars for cooking, a hundred if I'd be willing do it topless.

It's part of the reason I've got a stack of money in a safety deposit box in a downtown bank.

"Pasta primavera," I say and Alan snorts. His cough is deep, chronic, and he's given up both smoking and drinking, but he draws the line at meat. I'm trying to get him off it, thinking a better diet would steady his health. But he's eighty, and we both know nothing's going to help much at this point.

"Rabbit food," Alan says, poking a clump of broccoli.

"Next time, steak," he orders. I roll my eyes. We'll eat dinner together, I'll stack the plates in the sink, and before seven I'll be done.

I sit back and hug myself. My skin is clammy.

"Kinda cool in here," I say.

Tomorrow the earth will pass as close to the sun as it will all year. It's some unbelievable difference, like a million miles or something, so maybe I think it will be a particularly warm day.

"Put your sweater on," Alan says.

I shrug. I know he hardly cares about my tits anymore, but a deal's a deal.

In the morning I wake up to see my mother foraging though my closet. From the graying light outside my window I can tell it's about six. I slit my eyes half. My first class isn't until ten.

"Hey, uh-uh." I pipe up when I catch her trying on my leather jacket.

"Don't get up," she says. "It's still early." She swings my jacket back on a hanger, turns in front of the mirror in my new black jeans.

I sit up on my elbows. The jeans look pretty good on her. She's lost weight and recently had her hair cut short.

"Honey, can I borrow these? Or maybe you could pick up another pair." She reminds me of myself, as a kid, playing dress up in her closet. Then again, from the back, she looks so much like me right now. We are built the same, short waisted, all legs. She turns towards me. I sink back into bed.

"I'm off to work," she says. "Home late tonight. Your father's leaving soon."

My mother seems especially cheerful for someone I'd seen only hours ago sprawled out half wasted in front of a flickering TV. I had covered her with an afghan, a geometric white and black one my grandmother made. I left her there in our living room to sleep it off like a crumpled pop-art painting.

As I covered her up she mumbled, "I don't love your father. Elliot, I don't even trust him."

Twenty years ago my parents' wedding announcement made the *Times*. My father was a history professor, one of the youngest in an elite Ivy League school. He had been active in the civil rights movement and then had written his dissertation about voting rights. He had a beard and wore turtlenecks instead of suits and ties, and all of it shocked and displeased his parents who had brought him up amidst the who's whos of socialite Boston.

My mother was an undergraduate, studying to be the mathematician she eventually became ten years later.

They met at an anti-war rally where he was one of the speakers. He has a low, powerful voice — like his father, a successful courtroom lawyer — and though now my father is merely handsome, I have seen pictures of him from that time, and he was stunning.

The wedding announcement, which I looked up on the Microfiche in the university library, gave the basics of both families without color or depth, like those outlines in children's coloring books. This included the claim that my mother's father was born in Vienna and was in import-export. He actually owned a grocery on the Lower East Side that carried Chinese and Italian foods. That my grandmother was a homemaker was not worth mention, nor the fact that my mother was already pregnant with me.

If I didn't know better, I'd have read that announcement and said, "Hey, they did okay."

I do the house accounts. It started in high school. There was never food in the fridge, and one day the heat ran out because they forgot to order oil. So I just did it myself. I took the checkbook and signed my father's name, and it was as easy as that. By the end of my sophomore year I had a house ledger on my mother's computer and managed everything from the mortgage to the health insurance premiums to getting dog food for the dog that eventually ran away.

Now everything runs smoothly. Their pay checks and various dividends are automatically deposited into the account, and I skim a few hundred now and again as payment for my services. Actually quite often. Actually thousands a year more than my allowance.

Rhonda is my friend at college. Most of my high school friends went away somewhere else. I get to go here free because of my father. Not that we don't have the money to send me somewhere else. It just never came up when it was time to send out applications.

"Hey," Rhonda says. She is sitting at the far end of the second floor of the science library. It's where we always sit; we've even claimed the desks as our own. Rhonda has a picture of Bob Marley taped to hers. I've got this photo of these underwater animals called manatees on mine. They look like swimming cows. I like that they're so heavy but appear so light. I just found out there's this place in Florida where you can swim with them.

Rhonda's face is squinched up because she's concentrating on this piece of paper in front of her half covered with notes. Her dreads are almost to her shoulders now, and she's got this silver nose ring in her right nostril.

She's a history major. I met her last fall when I went to see my father at his office. She and I left the building at the same time. Rhonda said to me, "I hear he's always boffing one of his students. Black girls. This friend of my roommate got pregnant by him."

First I just stared at her and the words rolled right over me. I said, "So what." Then I started crying. She followed me to the bathroom and later, after I had stopped crying, I told her he was my father. She understands. Her dad has affairs, too.

"Potatoes are really great," Rhonda says smiling up at me. "They really have saved the world, you know. Because when people used to pillage places — like in Europe and everywhere — they sort of raped and plundered and took all the food, wheat and grain and stuff. So the people who had gotten away had nothing to come back to."

"So," I say, arranging myself at my desk. I've got a Diet Coke for each of us. Rhonda's got a bag of pistachios. "What's the point?" Professors are always asking you what's the point of things, and although Rhonda and I have discussed how the point usually isn't half as interesting as what is right in front of them, they still always want a point.

"*So*," she says, "once people started planting potatoes there was always food to come back to, because the plunderers didn't have time to dig 'em all up. So people could scatter without worrying and without having to drag sacks of grain and shit along with them. I'm calling it "The Potato — colon — Plotting the Development of Resistance."

Already Rhonda and I both know that you have to have a colon in the title of your paper if you want to get an A.

"Bravo," I say. "But nothing about young black wenches? He'll be disappointed." Rhonda has my father for European history. We try to make a joke of it.

I'm supposed to be writing this paper on an aspect of human evolution but I don't really have a topic yet. I read in one of the textbooks that vaginal contractions function to help sperm get to the egg quicker. This makes me think about how good lovers have a better chance of making babies. This makes me think about my father and that girl Rhonda told me about. I can just see the title: "Orgasms — colon — Giving Adulterers the Critical Edge."

"I'm going home for lunch," I say.

As I head out of the library I see my father by the admissions office. He's wearing a cap and is bent attentively towards a guy my age. He's supposed to be one of the best teachers on campus, may be in line to be the next department chair.

I go home for lunch but really to check the mail. Because there are certain envelopes addressed to my parents that I just don't want them to open. Turning up my street, I see my mother's Mazda in the drive. The red flag is still upright, though: The mailman hasn't come.

I can hear music from outside the house, new age stuff: lots of flutes and horns and those bouncy melodies that seem to me little more than audio Hallmark cards. There's hardly ever music in the house; it's a bad sign. I hesitate at the door, then enter making lots of noise. I hear my mother in the living room, laughing.

"Elliot," she calls. "Elliot? Is that you? Come in, there's someone here I'd like you to meet."

Reluctantly I turn into the large room. My mother looks up expectantly. She is set in the corner of the couch, knees tucked up underneath her like some schoolgirl. A man with thinning hair — maybe he's thirty, maybe a bit more — is wedged into the opposite corner of the couch. He's wearing tortoise-shell glasses and a ridiculous brown hand-knit tie that looks like the end of one of those dish towels you always find at church bazaars. He shifts to stand.

My mother moves over and rests her hand on his shoulder. The glass-top table is strewn with food: brie, a length of French bread, black olives, a bottle of wine, half empty.

"This is Doug. Doug, Elliot."

Doug looks puzzled. "Elliot," he says. "Well, after your mother mentioned an 'Elliot' I can honestly say I expected to meet a young man." His voice is puffed up and pompous like he's trying to be an adult. Meanwhile there are bread crumbs freckling his tie like scales of dandruff.

He's probably a graduate student, like the last guy that came around. That was about three months ago, and the guy actually did wear one of those plastic pen holders in his shirt pocket. I met him twice, the last time on the train when he and my mother were on their way home from a math conference out west. Then he disappeared.

I figured him a fluke, not the beginning of a pattern. Besides, I can't believe that my mother would go out with the kind of guys I turned down in high school.

"You're finishing your first year at the U?" he asks. I notice he's got one earring in his left ear, like that's going to save him from eternal nerdiness.

"Aren't you home early?" my mother interrupts.

"I forgot something," I say. "A book." But I'm thinking: *You're the one who said you'd be home late.*

I head up the stairs to my room. Once there I stare at myself in the mirror. My lips are chapped and there's the beginning of a cold sore on the top one, so it feels like it sticks out a mile. But you can't see it. After enough book search time, I tromp back down the stairs. As I come down I can hear my mother's animated voice explaining my name. "She was born the night after my father, Elliot, died. And don't you think —"

I poke my head in the door. "Nice to meet you." My mother's hand is now across the back of the couch. She's just had her nails done, moons of pastel pink.

"If you see your father, tell him I'll be late tonight."

I nod, resisting the urge to say, *Make sure you get home before midnight.*

Outside in the bright sunlight I'm relieved to find the mailman has come. There's the electric bill, a VISA statement and a long, fat envelope. Airline tickets. I tuck the envelope into the inside pocket of my backpack. I told Rhonda I'm taking her camping as soon as school is out. She's never been camping. She doesn't know we're going to be camping in Australia, then Bali.

But first we're stopping off in Florida, to swim with those manatees.

At Alan's I let myself in the back door. He sleeps in the afternoons, and sometimes I study there, even on nights I don't cook. I make myself coffee and spread my books on the table and then I hear his raspy cough coming from the sun porch.

"That you?" he says.

"Who else?"

I take my mug out to the porch. There's a funny smell, like camphor or mint, the smell of the gel he rubs on his chest when it bothers him.

He's half sitting up, a heavy blanket over his legs. There's a clipboard on the floor beside his bed, a yellow legal pad covered with writing and figures. I pick it up and scan the scribbles.

"Not bad. Eighty-four hundred." Alan plays along with "Jeopardy."

"Did you win?" I ask.

"No, some joker went double or nothing. The final category was Rock and Roll History. It's hardly history if you're my age. Anyway, I hadn't a clue."

Below the "Jeopardy" figurings are sentences. I skim them. "He held pivotal posts at . . . wrote numerous articles and books including . . . served in the United States Army as a captain . . ."

At the bottom of the page Alan wrote, "He is survived by," fragment leading nowhere.

All Alan's family is dead; he's been a widower for ten years, and his only son died in a car crash before I was born.

"What's this stuff?" I say. "The final 'Jeopardy' question, 'Who is Alan Reizenfeld?'"

He grabs the television clicker, his yellowed thumb pressing the volume button repeatedly. The TV stays on the whole day; the volume goes up and down. As the music to "Oprah" fades in, he says, "Thought I'd get my obit ready."

There's a mechanical pencil tucked into the top of the clipboard. After the words "survived by," I write "Elliot" on top of those three dots.

Oprah is about to talk to people who have fallen in love at first sight. This one woman says she and her fiancé locked eyes on the subway. The woman's hair is all blown up like cotton candy, and she's got a really strong New York accent.

"I'm asking Rhonda for dinner," I say and leave the room.

It's not one of my regular nights, but Alan doesn't care. The nights Rhonda comes we eat vegetarian stuff, and afterwards they play cards or sometimes chess. I never play games when there's no stakes, and Alan's got this rule of no gambling under his roof.

I never go topless when Rhonda's there, but still I get a clean hundred for the night. Alan and Rhonda enjoy themselves. I do, too.

VOWS

This week Alison has attended many social functions: a bridal shower, a mother/daughter bridal luncheon, and a wedding rehearsal followed by a formal dinner. Tonight she made an appearance at the bachelorette's party. A man dressed as a construction worker stripped to the screeching delight of Marion (her brother's fiancée) and her seven bridesmaids. Alison watched the stripper: obviously gay. Empathetic, she walked him to the door after the show.

"I'd rather be at the bachelor's party," he said, winking. Alison nodded. She could understand wanting to be somewhere else.

"What do they think," Leigh asks. "We don't sleep on sheets like the rest of the world? Or that we have a *phobia* about new appliances?"

Alison is talking on the phone with her lover Leigh, who is in their apartment in Los Angeles. Alison's mother and stepfather have just gone to bed and "Tonight Show" theme music leaks from under their bedroom door. Alison has just told Leigh about the box of used kitchen stuff her brother has passed on to her: Marion didn't want anything from Jim's first marriage in the new house.

"We could use some of that wedding loot," Leigh continues. "Silverware, a gleaming toaster —"

"I wish you were here," Alison cuts in.

"Don't start that again," Leigh says and they hang up soon after. Alison feels as if she's space walking and her co-pilot has just cut the cord.

It's just past three p.m. and so hot in St. Louis that Alison's pantyhose are stuck to her legs like flypaper. People arrive at the church in twos and threes. Alison is perched at the church entrance, behind a small table festooned with pale pink roses. From her vantage she can see one of her brother's ushers hunched over the steering wheel of his BMW sniffing from a small vial.

Alison shifts from one foot to the other, carefully balancing on the three-inch spikes strapped to her feet. Her blue-gray dress hits just below her knees, and her heels — not to mention her eyeshadow — match her dress perfectly. Wearing a strand of her grandmother's pearls, she looks not unlike many of the young attractive women who are fluttering up the church stairs.

Alison is smiling. At least she thinks she is, but her mother comes by to tell her it's more like a smirk.

"I'm trying," Alison replies. The wife of her brother's boss picks up the silver pen and signs in with a flourish.

"Thank you," Alison says. "The groom's side is to the left."

"You do look beautiful," her mother says. "Your hair looks nice like that."

This sounds like a compliment, but Alison knows what she's really saying: *For once you look like a girl.*

On a nearby table, silver and white boxes are stacked like children's building blocks. Alison's mother drifts back into the church and Alison continues to greet people automatically.

It's a second marriage for Jim, the first for Marion. They met less than a year ago on a blind date and within a month were engaged. Marion, a thirty-two-year-old frosted blonde, is a year younger than Alison. She's an only child, from a very well-to-do family. Jim's been trying to hitch up with someone for the last two years, ever since his first wife left him. This first wife fell in love with her therapist and is now living in England. But for some reason — pride? machismo? — Marion's parents think she is dead.

For the last three months Alison has fought with everyone — Jim, Marion, her mother and finally Leigh — about Leigh not being invited to the wedding. Even though she and Alison have been together eight years, Alison's stepfather still thinks Leigh is her "good friend" and her mother has repeatedly instructed her to keep him believing that. Nevertheless, Alison felt Leigh should have been invited regardless of the intimate details of their personal life. "It would seem funny," her mother said. "You bringing a *friend* all the way from California."

There were moments when Alison thought she was getting through to her mother, but then Jim or Marion would get to her mother between calls and she'd tow the line. "It would make Jim very unhappy," she finally confided to Alison.

Early on, Marion had asked Alison not to leak anything about her "lifestyle" to her folks. "My parents are very conservative," Marion explained. "They'll come around, but we have to give them some time to get to know you as *you*." Eventually, Leigh got sick of Alison's family and their crazy phone calls and said she wouldn't go even if they all begged "collectively and on their knees."

"You know how long it took *me* to understand it," her brother told her the night before the wedding. "Besides, Leigh probably wouldn't have enjoyed herself. It's a very dressy affair." Jim has only met Leigh twice and each time she was in jeans. Although he knows of her well-paid job as a hospital administrator, Jim probably imagines Leigh's entire wardrobe is denim.

People sign the guest book; some make polite inquiries about her life. "Not married yet?" asks Mabel Downs, the widow who has done her mother's perms ever since Alison was a little girl. "Better watch it, spinsterhood is just around the corner!"

Alison smiles, but this time she really does know it's a smirk.

Hank Stevens arrives scooting around the parking lot in his tiny sports car. An old college friend, Hank is Alison's escort for the day.

"Looking good," he says. They hug. Hank and his boyfriend still live in town and he's sacrificed this day to be her support. He's tall, well-built, easily one of the best looking guys in the hall. Alison sees her mom craning around and knows Hank's looks will please her.

The organist changes the tempo of the music, the cue for Alison to close the guest book. She and Hank march arm-in-arm up the aisle to the front pew. Alison tries to imagine she and Leigh walking up such an aisle but cannot get her mind to grasp the details: Who would wear what? What would they say? There are scattered whispers as she and Hank reach their seats.

After the service — short and traditional — everyone gathers in a large room where a band plays a string of what sound like Barry Manilow tunes. Drinks are flowing and Hank and Alison start in on champagne. Alison's brother gives Hank's hand a good strong pump, as though Hank may be the man to bring Alison around.

Marion approaches and pecks her on the cheek, a very intimate gesture given their relationship. "We're sisters now," Marion says, giggling. "Sisterhood is powerful," Alison replies without thinking. Marion looks at her quizzically.

Marion's mother arrives and looks Alison up and down. "Really, you are a very attractive young woman," she says. She fluffs Alison's hair which, despite gobs of hair goop and showers of hair spray, is beginning to wilt.

The first boy Alison ever kissed is one of her brother's attendants. "Ever?" asks Hank when she tells him. And as she assures him, he checks out the young man: blond streaked hair, tanned skin set off by a bright Hawaiian shirt. "It must have been memorable," he says raising an eyebrow.

"Nope," she counters. "Wet and sloppy." The boy, who is now a man and whose name is Tom, approaches and he and Alison exchange pleasantries. She introduces him to Hank as the band starts up a pedestrian version of "Moon River."

"Would you mind if we danced?" Tom puts his hand on Alison's shoulder but addresses this to Hank.

"I'd rather if *we* danced," Hank quips. "But if you insist, I'm used to rejection." Tom stands there, unsure of what has happened. Alison rolls her eyes at Hank and pulls Tom onto the dance floor.

By five-thirty most everyone is plastered, including Alison. She hardly ever drinks and everything — champagne, fatigue, frustration — has gone to her head where it has joined to form a pounding salsa band. In the bathroom, she sits on the toilet for what seems like hours. She's exhausted. Her nerves are shot. She thinks of Leigh.

Leigh is wonderful, she thinks, perfect. Drunk, Alison is weepy and sentimental. She vows to finally forgive Leigh's last fling, with that country-western crooner she met at aerobics.

Alison is sniffling, still seated on the toilet, when there's a knock on the cubicle door. She peeks under the door. Shell-pink pumps. Her mother. "Hold on," she calls under the door. Rolling off her damp pantyhose, she smooths her dress down as best she can.

"Oh, *Al-i-son*." Her mother exhales dramatically when she exits the cubicle. "I've been wondering where you'd gone to. Hank's at the bar thwarting advances from every unattached woman in the hall."

"Their loss," Alison mumbles.

"You look a fright," her mother says. "Freshen your make-up."

Alison stands in front of the mirror. *Yes,* she thinks, *for once I agree with my mother: I do look a fright.*

Her mother grabs a paper towel, dampens the corner and dabs at Alison's face, under her eyes. Alison pulls away.

"I'm so tired of this," she says to her mother. "All these charades." Her eyes start to tear and she wipes her nose with the back of her hand.

The door opens and Marion's mother walks in. "Oh," she says, "is something the matter?"

"She's just feeling a little sick," Alison's mother places her hand on Alison's forehead. "Hot," she adds.

"Sick of all this," Alison says. Both women look at her. Both are wearing pastel dresses. The gladioli pinned to their bosoms reek. Alison is indeed nauseous.

"Sick of all this crap."

Marion's mother starts to retreat. "I'll leave you two to sort this out," she says crinkling her nose to punctuate her condescension. The stress of pulling together this social event has made everyone edgy. The women have been worrying for months about the details of this gala event and now that it is just about over, they are letting down their hair just a bit. Marion's mother starts to back out the door.

"No, wait! I'm —" Alison's voice breaks. Taking a deep breath, she starts again. "I'm gonna bring her to his *next* wedding, goddamn it . . ." The woman nods blankly at Alison and then, in confusion, glances towards her mother.

"I live with her, you know! I love her!" Alison adds, desperately, futilely.

Marion's mother shrugs, then disappears through the swinging door. Alison turns to her mother in the vain hope of finding recognition. Instead, she gets a slap across her face. Not hard, but she's never been hit by her mother before.

"You're not the only one in this family," her mother says.

They stare at each other. Alison's cheek buzzes like a limb waking up from sleep.

"Warts and all," her mother says finally breaking the staring spell. "Warts and all." This is her stepfather's answer to her mother's complaints meaning, *You get the good with the bad. We're all in this together.*

"I'm *not* a wart, " Alison says. "I mean, I'm —" Alison shakes her head. The salsa band starts up again. Everything she says sounds crazy.

Mabel Downs swings open the bathroom door. Alison's mother manages a weak smile, yet Mabel is not looking at their faces.

"You both need a good spray," she says and pulls a can of Final Net from her purse.

"I try," her mother mumbles quietly, and leaves the bathroom.

"It's not your fault, honey," Mabel says. "It's this damn heat."

Hank is at the bar chatting up the bartender. He and Alison leave without fanfare and drive to a nearby steak house. Alison walks in carrying her heels but no one seems to mind. She has sobered up some and has filled Hank in on the details — or at least those she can remember — of what she now refers to as the "Bathroom Bathos."

"At least they let you come to the damn thing," Hank says. "Last time I talked to my sister, I told her I was thinking about dropping in on the folks this summer. My mother called the next day and said she'd heard I was threatening to visit! *Threatening* — that's the word she used."

Alison is listening, but she's also trying to figure things out. Most likely nothing will change. Jim and Marion will go on their honeymoon; her mother will pretend like nothing ever happened. Tomorrow she'll fly home.

"And when my sister visited last year she wouldn't let her kids drink out of my glasses," Hank adds.

A blond waitress interrupts to ask Hank if he would like to order wine. He orders a beer, and she adds, "And something for the lady?"

The waitress smiles wide at Hank, assuming he's the tipper. Hank looks over at Alison.

"Lay off him," Alison says. "He's gay and anyway I'm paying. Queer as a three dollar bill. A faggot."

Hank stares. Then he adds, after a pause, in his best *sotto* voice, "So, *she's* a dyke." Hank loves games.

"Poofter!" Alison says.

"Lezzie!"

The waitress follows this short volley with her head as though watching championship tennis. Her eyebrows wrinkle and the smile melts from her face.

Hank and Alison begin laughing, quietly, then uncontrollably. The waitress, who has been watching with her pen poised, leaves.

Alison grabs Hank's hand across the table just as her laughter starts to crack. She bites her lower lip to keep from crying.

"I'm hungry," she says after a moment. "Now we'll never get anything to eat."

Hank squeezes her hand and turns to spot the waitress. "She's spying on us from behind that fern."

Alison tries to wave her over. "I'm sorry," she calls. "We're okay, really."

"We're *more* than okay," Hank says.

"Sure," Alison says, turning to face him. "But who would know it?"

ODDS ARE

Other families go to Yellowstone, or Mexico, or the Grand Canyon. We're going to Soledad, the prison, where my brother is, and we're all going to stay in a trailer for two days. What they call a family visit. I haven't told anyone, not even Myrna, my best friend. It's a pretty heavy place. There are murderers and rapists and all sorts of guys in there. I'm not sure I even want to go but Mom would die if I didn't. She's been cooking for days and the back of the pick-up is piled with bags and coolers full of Tom's favorite foods, too much for anyone to eat in two days. I made him cookies. Chocolate chip.

But I didn't feel like baking him cookies, and I didn't even lick the bowl afterwards. I'm five days overdue. I might be pregnant. I haven't told Glenn I'm late because I don't really want to think it's true, and I don't want to get into a whole hassle with him. He's Catholic, and I think he'd want me to have it. I'm not in love with him and I can't even remember if we had a good time that night.

Up till now I've been the only normal person in this family. The good one, somehow different from the others like if they were adopted. But just when everything starts to feel like things are getting right again for all of us, I had to do it just that once without my diaphragm because I thought I had counted the days right. About every five minutes I go to the bathroom and check for blood.

Mom thinks I've got the runs.

We left Anaheim when it was still dark. My mom driving and smoking and not saying anything. We live not too far from Disneyland and I could see the lights on the top of the Matterhorn as we turned onto the freeway. I used to have my birthday parties there when I was a kid, but then everyone did, and it was no big deal. When my father left and we had to move, I asked if we could go live there, on Main Street or in a log cabin on Tom Sawyer's island. I was five. Disneyland seemed like a great place to live.

After my dad left, we moved to this little pink house: my mother, my brother, me and the dog. Mom got a job as a checker at the Safeway. Turned out my brother didn't stick around long so Mom and I didn't have to share a bedroom. He's seven years older than me. I've suspected I was a mistake but I've never asked. I don't think it's anything I want to know for sure. But then sometimes I think my brother was the mistake — that he's why they got married. I don't know. The whole thing makes me sick to think about right now. At least I hope that's what's making me nauseous and not you-know-what.

My mom's pretty happy about this trip. She said, It's time this family got to be a family, and I thought to myself: *Yeah, right.* But then other than this lateness — which is what I'm calling it until I know, really know — things have been going okay. Okay for us that is.

My brother's due to get out of prison in two months. He's in there for a bunch of stuff mostly to do with drugs. I don't really know what happened because he got busted almost three years ago and I was only twelve. I've got this newspaper clipping that says murder and kidnaping and conspiracy but I think none of that came down in the end. He plea bargained and so he never went to trial, just jail. He went cold turkey there, and my mom said that saved his life. I don't really know him too well. I'm not sure I want to. He might be a murderer. One Easter, at this egg hunt sponsored by the Jaycees, he gave me all his eggs. I don't think a murderer is that kind of guy but I don't know.

And my mom. She just had her one year birthday, in the program that is. A.A. Alcoholics Anonymous. She used to drink a lot. I never knew before if it was a real lot because it was how she always drank. It's like with Myrna, she has this birthmark right under her chin, next to her left ear. I'm so used to it I don't even see it. But then we'll go into a shop to try on make-up or something and the lady will always ask what happened to her, like if she was burned or something. And then I see it again, all red and splotchy. It was the same thing with my mother's drinking.

So Mom's got this chip thing now, hanging on her key chain

and twisting from the dashboard, proving that she's been one year sober and things are really a whole lot better at home. She's gone a lot, at meetings, but when she's at home she's *there*, not like before. Once or twice I went to Ala-teen just to see what it was like, but then I felt like I was above those kids. You know, like I wasn't a screw-up. Now look who's talking.

The Hansens: Tom's getting sprung soon, Mom's going to be promoted to assistant manager at the Safeway and she's pretty happy seeing this Martin guy from the program. And then there's me. Good grades, I don't do drugs, but now there's this.

Sometimes I smoke. Cigarettes.

We drove up 101 and the sun came up somewhere around Santa Barbara. The ocean was flat with fog melting into the pale blue sky like steam off hot soup. I asked Mom to stop, so she pulled over at the city beach. While I went to the bathroom to check she skimmed rocks along the shore line. She's actually decent looking, my mom, when she wears nice clothes. She's slim with brown hair cut in a bob above her ears. I don't even think she's forty yet. I came out of the bathroom as she walked up the beach.

"What's the story, morning-glory?" she said. She smiled and tried to bop me on the ear. I pulled away. I think she sometimes doesn't realize how old I am.

"Can I drive?" I wanted to think of something else besides getting my period.

"You know how to?"

I'm fifteen and of course I don't have a license, but I've been driving forever, mostly on dates when guys get too drunk. It looked like she was almost willing to let me, but then she said no, and I slid over.

"I'll bet there's a lot of things you can do that I don't know about," she said and got behind the wheel.

"No," I said. "Probably not."

"Betcha," she said.

Ha.

"I've got a surprise for you and Tom," she said as we left Santa Barbara behind.

"What?"

"A big surprise."

46

I looked out the window thinking, *just what I need*. She looked at me and put her hand across the back of the seat and then on my shoulder.

"Hey," she said, and I looked at her. "It's a good surprise, it really is." She turned her eyes back to the road. "A great surprise."

The idea of a good surprise is pretty hard to figure. And at this point in my life I'm not sure if I can be surprised at all.

"But I'm not going to tell you until we're all together."

In September, the inside of California is pretty dry and empty. Everything was different shades of brown: the mountains, the hills, the fields which had just been cleared for winter. Sometimes there were patches of wildflowers, pinpricks of yellow and purple. For a while we drove behind a truck piled with tomatoes, and each time there was a bump in the road a few slipped over the edge and bounced to the shoulder. There were other vegetables on the high-way; I saw artichokes, lettuce, even a cauliflower. My mom said it looked like Safeway's produce department on a bad day.

We passed a few towns and some small cities. I wondered what it would be like to live in the sticks. I wondered what the kids were like there. Somehow I think the families in those towns aren't like mine. I'm sure they're not. Kids in those kinds of places ride horses. Still, I'll bet the high school girls screw around as much as anywhere else.

Most of the way Mom played tapes. One-day-at-a-time stuff — from the program. They've got these slogans: Let Go and Let God, Live and Let Live. Each one of those got stuck in my head for at least sixty miles. I slipped my finger into my pants every once in while; hunger can make you feel like you're getting your period.

It was afternoon by the time we got to Soledad. And it was hot. Before the town and before you reach the prison there's this billboard: "It's Happening in Soledad." For real. With a rainbow and everything painted right on it. Mom stopped the car to take a snapshot for Tom, and I went behind one of those round desert bushes to pee. Mom told me that Soledad meant solitude in Spanish.

The prison looked like a huge rat cage, a big box ringed by chain-link fences higher than goal posts with barbed wire wrapped like moss around everything. Inside the fence a whole bunch of white guys were sitting in the sun with their shirts off. Some black guys were playing basketball. I squinched my eyes so I couldn't see the fence and it looked like any schoolyard on a Sunday afternoon.

It took hours for us to be checked out. They went through all the food, all our clothes. One guard flirted with me, and I was friendly because I didn't know if he might get down on Tom if I wasn't. Three other women were there to see their husbands. They were really dressed up, especially this one black woman who had really high heels. She could barely balance on them. One lady had a baby.

Finally, we were shown through to a row of trailers. There were four and ours was one in the middle. Tom was waiting at the door.

"Welcome to Club Fed," he said and threw his arms out wide. He looked heavier than I had ever seen him, even a belly out in front. But then the last time I saw him he was pumping heroin.

Mom ran to hug him and he picked her up off the ground. I looked around, and everyone else was making out at the door of their trailers. Even the woman with the baby. It was on the ground with its feet kicking in the air. The trailers were partitioned from the bigger prison by a net of wire but some guys were on the other side watching and hooting.

"Go for it, V-man" one yelled. The guy next door waved to him and then slung his wife over his shoulder and went into the trailer.

"Looking good," Tom said to me. I didn't know what to say. I hadn't seen him in two years.

"I have a surprise for you," my mother said. Her eyes were wet and glassy. "A big surprise," she said and hugged him again.

A guard put our stuff in the trailer and moved back through the double wired gates that surrounded the small yard. He winked at me on his way out.

"Your sister's a fox," one guy shouted through the fence and another guy whistled. Tom flipped them off and we all went inside.

I ate about a million calories that night. We played poker and pinochle. Every three hours a bell would go off and Tom would have to go out and report. A guard looked in his eyes a couple of times, I guess to figure out if he was drinking or taking anything.

The trailer was small, with a small living area and kitchen and two tiny bedrooms. It felt like there were too many of us in the room. A wisp of breeze came in through the little screened windows but the desert air was warm. Other than bidding and dealing Tom didn't say much. My mother was bugging me. I think she was bugging Tom, too. She kept talking about A.A., and then flirting with her surprise. She talked about it all night and always with a voice like she was announcing the winner of a supermarket sweepstakes.

"So tell us already," Tom said after she'd said it about a hundred times. "Tell us about your damn surprise." He lit a cigarette and threw the pack at me. I pulled one out but didn't light it. I didn't think he had to be so mean. It was like he pulled a chair out from under her or something.

Still holding her cards fanned out in front of her, she pushed back her chair. "I tried my best," she said. "I really tried." She sounded fragile and cracked, and I waited for her to cry. She set her cards on the edge of the table and they toppled onto the floor. I could hear noises from the trailer next door. A lady giggling.

"It's okay, Mom," I said. I felt bad for her. Tom just sat there and smoked. "What's your surprise?"

"It doesn't matter."

"No, tell us," I said.

"Tom doesn't care."

"He does too."

"No, he doesn't."

"You do care, don't you Tom?"

"Sure," he said, but not like he did. I stared at him. Really stared. I mean this wasn't our dream vacation. Mom hid her face in her hands.

"I do care," he said and then the bell went off for him to go outside. "I do care," he said, softer, before leaving.

Mom went into the little bathroom and washed her face. I played with the cigarette and felt my underwear. After a while Tom came back in. Mom started washing some dishes. I watched them both, not sure of what to do, feeling almost invisible.

"I'm pregnant," Mom said above the dishes. "I'm going to marry Martin, and we'll all move to his house in Huntington."

I looked at Tom. He was lying on his back on the small green couch, smoking. His face didn't change, not a bit.

"We're going to be a family again," she said. "We have another chance."

No one said anything for a long time. Finally I went outside. The people next door were sitting on their porch and they waved at me. I waved back, neighbor-like. I sat on our picnic table. I thought about moving. I didn't want to, but I couldn't really figure out why not. I thought I could maybe live with Myrna so I wouldn't have to change schools. Not that my school was so great.

Tom came out wearing only boxer shorts. The lights in our trailer went out. The yard was still bright because of the search lights on the patrol towers.

"So," he said. "Are you surprised by the surprise?"

"No," I said, although I may have been.

He offered me a cigarette and we smoke there, like two adults. The warm air made a faint whistling sound as it blew through all the wire and fences. I could see a dark face up in the tower closest to us. I wondered where my father was. Whether he had other kids now, what they were like. There were a lot of things I didn't know.

"Did you kill someone?" I asked finally.

"What if I said I did?" I didn't say anything. Would I feel differently about him, or feel anything at all?

"I didn't," he said without looking at me.

We sat there for a while. Tom lit two more smokes and offered me one. "Don't you believe me?" he said.

"I think so."

Does it matter?"

"Yes, it does," I said because that was what seemed to matter right then. Not Mom's baby or Martin or even a baby of mine, but whether Tom was a murderer or not. Things suddenly started to break up in my head like if someone had turned on a blender in my brain.

Tom was looking up at the stars. You could see them even through the halo of searchlights. I looked around for a moon and couldn't find one.

"Mom deserves something good," Tom said. "She'll get to start over."

My stomach felt strange, maybe from the cigarettes, but it felt like my period. Right then Tom seemed like an okay person.

50

We smoked the whole pack and Tom went inside and got another. Later in the night I asked him about our dad and he said he was a bastard. Then he said no, he was a nice enough guy. Only that he wasn't very nice to Mom.

The bell went off once during the night and the guys in the other trailers stumbled out and waved to the man in the tower. One didn't have any clothes on. Tom just stayed sitting on the table.

"That guy killed someone," he said. It was the guy who had waved to me.

I thought I felt cramps but I didn't run to check. I figured if my mother was pregnant, odds were I wasn't.

We sat there all night. The air cooled off much later. It must have been four or five because not long after that it started to get light. It happened quickly, or maybe I was so tired I didn't notice it creeping up. It was like someone had lit a match in back of the mountains. A glow came up from behind them, and with it a warmth. As the stars faded out, it felt like the world was starting over.

Monuments

The day before we left on this vacation I came home from work and found the telephone book opened to Sperm Banks. There were three listings, one within walking distance. There were also pencil scratchings on the page: Elsie's doodling, a mixture of arrows and spirals, like a small treasure map. There were some numbers in the margin: maybe hours, maybe prices. Maybe even an appointment time.

Elsie is thirty-five years old and she wants a baby now. And I'm not sure I do. If she hadn't brought it up I certainly wouldn't have. Elsie is going to do it, she says, with me or without me.

"Oh my god, Kate," is what Elsie says. It's an understatement but it's probably the same thing I would say if I could say anything at all. I am speechless. I drive the car five miles an hour. My head wags side to side like a carnival puppy. After days of hellish driving, not to mention nights of hellish camping, we have arrived at Mount Rushmore.

There are motorcycles parked ten deep in the parking lot. Cars are frantically trying to weave in and out of narrow parking spaces made narrower by gleaming hunks of steel which have sidled in beside each vehicle like some sort of parasites. The grassy areas between the lots are covered with motorcycles, and so is the shoulder of the blistery two-lane road. The sound of bike engines drowns out our tape of new age Muzak. Between the bikes, on the bikes, and pouring towards the multicolored flags at the entrance to the park, are swarms of black-clad bodies. It looks like an ant farm in the midst of an industrial revolution.

I drive cautiously to the entrance of the last lot and a pimply and sunburned kid points me to an available space. He looks apologetic, I think, or perhaps it's the heat. Elsie is laughing. This is not my idea of a holiday — *uh, uh* — and, no, I am not laughing. Mount Rushmore was Elsie's idea and therefore it only strikes me as a little odd that she is laughing, now, so hard that tiny rivulets of water are tracking the wrinkles at the corners of her eyes. In light of last night it is pretty funny.

Last night we camped at the O-Kee-Doe-Kee Korral which was listed in our Triple-A guidebook as a "perfect place for family camping." We pitched our tent next to a miniscule trickle of water — the advertised "river" — and just after the sandman had paid us a visit, we were neighbored by a batch of noisy bikers swinging six-packs. They roared up on huge choppers like a swarm of motorized locusts. Elsie fell back to sleep immediately. They proceeded, as they say, to "party." I tossed and turned, wanted to leave, thought of going to the manager. Woke Elsie up twice with these ideas. Finally I stuffed my ears with some cotton that I found in Elsie's makeshift first-aid kit. Even then it was a rocky sleep. When we pulled out this morning I yelled "Good riddance!" at their sleeping-bagged bodies. One guy peeked over the top of his bag, a white face framed by a mass of strawberry blonde hair. Elsie called "Have a nice day!" and laughed.

And now she's really laughing. Because here at Mount Rushmore there are bikers *everywhere*. Elsie goes to talk with the parking kid. I am standing behind the Honda, drawing snake designs in the coat of dust that covers the rear window. "WASH ME," I write because I know it will make Elsie giggle. As she crosses the parking lot towards me I rub it off and write "KISS ME" underneath.

"You won't believe it," she says.

"What?" I wipe the KISS ME off, too, and the heel of my hand is covered in red dirt.

"The Twentieth Annual Harley Davidson Rodeo and Round-up," she says, waving towards the end of the lot where most of the bikes are parked. "Here. Now. This entire weekend. Sixty thousand bikers." We both smile. "A big old party," she says and laughs a very Elsie laugh. Last night I almost had her convinced that we should change camp sites; I was certain there would be quiet at the next one.

"Wonder what Lincoln thinks of black leather?" she asks, and we gather up our cameras and join the snake of pedestrians weaving towards the mount.

This trip is a compromise, a test, a beginning or an ending, but none of it has gone the way I'd thought it would go. I'm not outdoorsy — my idea of an adventure is to set out on a holiday without motel reservations. For years we have vacationed separately; sometimes I go to Cannes for the films, Monterey for the jazz. Mostly I spin work-perks into free urban vacations. I work for the morning daily, my by-line: Kate Perkins, Staff Critic. Elsie generally takes camping trips with girlfriends from the high school where she teaches, or with people from her political affinity group. Last year she went to Nicaragua on a work brigade. I admire her spirit and commitment. She appreciates my intellect, my humor. We've been together ten years now — living together for five.

I met Elsie at a club in San Francisco, at a punk rock show I was reviewing. She looked bright and cheerful, not like the usual punk girl, sullen and serious. When we met I told her I was a reviewer — to impress her — and she laughed in my face. "So who does that make you?" she asked, and I told her my name, thinking *then* she would be impressed. She laughed again. Spunky.

Elsie doesn't believe in reviewers, thinks most of what we write is a subjective crock of shit, and being with me these past ten years has failed to convince her otherwise. She's got spine, approaches everything and everybody with a clean slate. Even if something's a runaway favorite, she makes it prove itself to her. That's a good critic. I'm good, but I tell you every time I take her along I get something from her. "Behind every woman . . ." Elsie says after she whispers something in my ear at a performance, "there's another woman telling her what to write." Quite often she's right.

I had the club beat for years, but now they've got someone younger than me to write about music: He's young, he's hip, with jeans so tight you can see the tendons flex behind his knees. I'm forty and even if I was interested in going to the clubs (which I'm not), forty is a bit old to be a pop music critic. I've paid my dues and now my editor generally lets me write on pretty much whatever I want. I've just finished a slightly academic book about drugs and music which may, if not make me money, put me on the talk show circuit.

Anyway, I like my job. I'm even out there. But is this enough? Is this a life? This is what Elsie has asked. Because Elsie wants a baby.

We've gotten down to the grit with this question. If I don't want to have a child, fine, she says. She'll find something to inseminate with (turkey baster or otherwise) and move out and we can still be friends. Maybe even lovers. But she is pretty determined. For months I've found magazine clippings around the apartment, articles about artificial insemination and diet during pregnancy. Somehow these seemed totally abstract until I saw that list of sperm banks. Elsie is very ethical: If I don't want a kid she's not going to bring one into our home. But — here's the catch — she's going to find a new home.

"Unbelievable," she says. I don't know if she's talking about the crowd or the mountain. Is it sculpture? What else can you call it? We are standing on the observation platform with hundreds of black-clad bikers and nearly an equal number of white American families. There are Asian tourists scattered between. All groups are trying to ignore each other; yet I think more people are checking out everybody else than are admiring the guys carved into the side of the mountain.

But Elsie is staring at the mountain, and it is unbelievable. It's huge and daunting and yet laughable. She turns to me and rolls her sea-green eyes. "Patriotic and patriarchal," she says. "I guess Bobo Walker was right."

In part I can thank Bobo Walker for this trip. Bobo Walker is poor and black and is in Elsie's tenth grade American history class. He's unmotivated and gets into trouble, but Elsie believes he is very gifted. One day she was showing slides and Bobo was fooling around with one of the girls in the back of the room. There was a slide of Rushmore on the screen. Elsie asked Bobo to identify the slide: "Four white dudes in rock, big fuckin' deal." The class busted up and Elsie said "Yes, Bobo, I guess you've got a point there." She came home from school that day tired, as always, and proposed this Americana vacation. "I have to figure out why I'm teaching this stuff," she said. She cares, really cares about those kids. And every scratch of writing on the wall suggests she'd be an excellent parent.

Elsie and I take seats on the observation deck, and a family plops itself down next to us. The kids confirm my worst suspicions about this generation of children. "Hey, Elsie," I shoot my eyes left to where they are seated so that she will look, too. She glances at them briefly, then buries herself in a guide book.

The parents are no older than Elsie and me. Dad is wearing green slacks, a yellow and red striped polo shirt, a rainbow of color spun from the L.L. Bean catalogue. His hair is cropped à la Ollie North. The woman wears that washed-out look of modern motherhood. She's not unattractive — a jogger, I imagine. Frosted hair under a pale purple visor, a pink t-shirt and pastel running shoes. I compare her to Elsie: red flaming hair and curvy hips wrapped in tight, torn Levi's; the oddly-shaped Birkenstock sandals that remind me of the boats I carved out of bark as a child.

This man and woman hardly talk. The boy and girl, looking very much like miniature versions of their parents, jabber nonstop. Mostly complaints. They hate this kind of ice cream, it's too hot, can't they go swimming at the hotel? Then a gang of bikers walks past, older and weathered. One has a pony-tail, looped with a faded red bandanna, that snakes down the center of his back.

"Disgusting," says the girl as they pass. "They're so gross." She looks all of about thirteen and she pulls out a thin tube of lipstick from her white hip-slung purse and coats her lips with shell-pink frosting.

"They *smell*," says the boy, louder, so that I am sure the men can hear. I am embarrassed yet I look to see if the parents will give a lecture on tolerance, or manners, or something. Instead they just follow the retreating men with their eyes and nod. I sneer, hoping the kids will see me, but they all get up and saunter off towards the parking lot.

I turn back to Elsie. I raise my eyebrows.

"I know what you're thinking," she says. "So what?"

"Hey," I say, trying to stop her.

"So they're creepy right-wing kids with creepy right-wing parents. So what?" There is a tinge of anger in her voice. She scans the observation deck dramatically. "Shall I find a couple of progressive, polite kids and point them out to you?" A tiny smile cracks the corners of her mouth. She waits until I smile, too, before returning to her guidebook. She's a hard one.

Elsie proposes that we split up and meet back in an hour. She wants to go see the history presentations and the slide show; I'm content to watch the bikers, many of whom genuinely seem interested in the four white dudes. Elsie skips off down the slope towards the sculptor's studio, and I watch her go. She's beautiful, sparkly and solid.

Right before she turns the bend into the trees she runs into a wall of black leather. Disentangling herself from the mass of shiny skins, she flashes her bright broad smile at the three men. They laugh, together. Even in her all-cotton clothing, it almost looks as if she is with them. The four of them walk off together down the path to the museum. Elsie is walking between two of them.

The gift shop is hopping and I walk through in a daze. There are the expected items: postcards, pennants, t-shirts, paperweights. But there are also such things as Rushmore nail clippers, Rushmore sheets, and chopping blocks with the faces of Rushmore on the surface. I consider buying one of these for Bobo Walker and then find out they want a whopping $12.95 for them, and they're not even real wood. I begin to select postcards: for my work buddies, my mother, and for Amanda. Amanda is a critic who works for the rival paper. We had an affair three years ago, I think mainly to find out the dope on each other's editors. She was curious about the whole girl thing. Anyway, we are friends now, she's engaged to be married, and she even comes to dinner occasionally. Elsie will eat with us but she won't cook those nights. "I'll eat with almost anyone," she says, "but there's no reason to cook for a gal who slept with my *woman.*" She overdramatizes this announcement every time Amanda comes over, as if she's threatening a showdown. But once together she and Amanda chat away. I suspect they are really better pals than Amanda and me.

"Honey," I hear and look up from the circular postcard rack automatically. It's not Elsie but a young woman in hip-high black boots and a black halter top. She's blonde and actually pretty. Her bronze heart-shaped face scans the area behind my right shoulder. I turn to see a hulk of a man, bearded, wearing a tattered leather jacket, worn jeans and a black mesh tank top. His hair is cropped short, his beard rests on his chest. His belly's the size of a good Sunday roast.

"Here I am, sweetie," he says and sidles around me so his hand rests on her hip.

"Doncha think this one would be great for Mother?" I try to see what card she is holding. It's one of those comic kind, with a jack-a-lope. He nods at her choice and pecks her on the ear. I turn in embarrassment, grabbing a stack of the card closest to me: "An Aerial View of Mount Rushmore." I pass the couple on my way to the register and I see a tattoo on the woman's right shoulder: "Property of Wiley Jones." It shocks me: so permanent, so prominent. I look at the man again. I wonder if his name is Wiley.

I'm bored. There are people swarmed in around me. Big ones. Little ones. Littler ones.

So Elsie wants a child. She knows this, and she came to know this as suddenly as if she'd been struck by lightning. Biological clock, she said. Biological time-bomb, I countered.

Before the last couple of years I never thought much about what I wanted. I had a good job; I loved Elsie. I've never been one to think about the future. There are books to write and places to go. I came of age at that time when commitment was a dirty word. Remember Free Love? Okay, so it wasn't free, and maybe it wasn't even love. But it's how the game was played.

In our own meandering way, Elsie and I have managed a lot longer than most of our friends. Our agreement has been to honesty, not necessarily commitment. And although we've both transgressed here and there over the years, at some point it became obvious to both of us that we're in this for the long haul. But a baby? Nighttime feedings? P.T.A.? Little League? A *teenager* — sex and drugs and rock 'n' roll? Elsie says I've got to have someone to dedicate my books *to*.

A little Elsie scampering around the apartment? Or a boy with a little willy out front? At times it does sound fun. Times like Christmas which I imagine — or hope — would be a whole lot more enjoyable with children. (Although our friends Jackie and Brett would disagree: They stayed up till three a.m. last Christmas Eve assembling a Barbie doll house and in the morning all little Crissy said was "You bought the wrong one!") Mostly, children sound like a terrible responsibility. I leaf through my list of glib but nonetheless reasonable excuses: the decline of the schools, the greenhouse effect, nuclear war. Elsie says to these: "So what? What else is a life?" And she adds, "My mother had me right after Hiroshima." I tell her, "I'm still a kid myself." She answers, "Good, then it'll have someone to play with." What of the kids in elementary school chirping "Your mothers are dykes" to our little protégé? "They say that to all kids." She's got an answer to everything.

So far I've skirted the subject as much as possible, which is partly why I've been so cranky. It's either that or the air mattress which, because of certain popped bubbles, makes me feel as though I'm sleeping on an opened egg carton. I know that tomorrow we'll start back home and that by the weekend I will have had to make some decision. I try out new vocabulary. The nouns "daughter" and "son" take on a whole new meaning with the addition of a certain pronoun. "My daughter," I mumble, "my son."

The kid sitting next to me looks up at me like I'm crazy. He's got ice cream running from the corners of his mouth, his high-top tennis shoes are laced in such a way that I cannot figure out how he gets them on or off. I shake my head, and then I catch myself. It's probably what my mother did when she saw me wearing love beads.

I look back at the monument.

Am I alone not enough for Elsie?

It's been an hour. I keep glancing at the mountain. It really is impressive; despite all that stone, it's graceful. The faces have affect; the eyes seem alive. I take several pictures of the mountain, then a couple of the bikers. One picture is perfectly framed. Four burly, rusty-headed men are standing against the rail directly below the carving looking in towards the deck. Their faces echo those of the presidents.

I decide to head towards the studio, to find Elsie. I want to show her the four men against the wall. She would love the composition.

I miss her.

Inside the building a young brunette is speaking in the tour-talk way. Behind her are photographs: scaffolds hundreds of feet high, tiny men resting against Washington's nostril, sticks of dynamite in their hands. I don't see Elsie in the full room. I back out the door and head for the parking lot; I can't quite remember where we said we would meet. The deck, I thought, but maybe the car.

She is not at the car. I walk back to the deck. It is not like Elsie to be late.

I am tired and hot and I trot back down the path to the studio. Elsie is still nowhere to be seen. The same ranger is talking.

"Gutzon Borglum was patriotic, fiercely so," says the perky ranger. "And he dreamed he was creating at Rushmore an everlasting symbol of the American dream, as well as his own ticket to immortality."

I am about slip out again when this word gets stuck in my ear. "Immortality." I think of my writing. Immortal? Hardly. I walk over yesterday's reviews cluttering the sidewalks on my way to work.

"Borglum died before he could see the work completed," she continues. "But his son, Lincoln, who worked with him much of his life, saw the project to completion." She pauses, "Any questions?"

I think of my father, a construction foreman. I cannot even imagine working with him, let alone finishing his life's work. He's hardly talked to me since 1968 when he found me smoking dope in the basement and listening to Canned Heat's "Amphetamine Annie" full blast with my arms around Cindy Thompson. He doesn't understand my work and has never read any of it, but once he told me his favorite film was *The Deer Hunter*. "A man's film," he said. He told my mother he thinks I will die young. "The girl's never sweated a day in her life," he said. He himself is a chipper sixty-nine. I feel unbearably hot. I want to escape both the room and the memories of my father. What makes me think we could do any better?

Back outside I start to think Elsie has been kidnaped. I wonder if what I have been told about bikers just might be true, that they are taking my Elsie to their camp where they will gang-rape her and make her cook sausages and eggs. It's a stupid fear, but I'm tired and scared, and I can't imagine why I can't find her.

She wouldn't, would she? In the woods? With a biker?

She wouldn't. But it's been two hours.

I decide to check the car once more before reporting her missing. I imagine the announcement: "Elsie Greenfield, thirty-five, red hair, green eyes, last seen wearing jeans and a light blue t-shirt with the words 'Women's Revolutionary Knitting Circle' stenciled across the front. Full hips," I hear, "child-bearing hips . . ." I skip down the stairs, past the multicolored flags of all the states and towards the car but I can't see anyone near it. My eyes are watering, from the wind and heat I think, but somehow I suspect tears all the same.

I am about to turn around and head back when I see a sliver of red on the bright green grass behind the Honda.

My heart crumbles.

I stop running, winded, and walk slowly towards the car. The tears are coming now, and I can't stop them. My gut is sucked into my ribs with each breath.

Elsie is sleeping on the grass next to the car, her hands are open at her sides, her face is slack and open to the sun. Freckles have crowded onto the bridge of her nose. There are small birds eating from a torn sack of trail mix that lies open near her hip. As I approach, they fly. And she opens her eyes.

"Honey," she says, slowly, drowsily. "I fell asleep." Her eyes flutter open momentarily. "I looked all over for you," she adds. Her eyes are closed again. "Where were you?"

She rolls herself over to face me; it is the same way she turns towards me in bed.

There have probably been more responsible reasons to have a baby, but there have also been worse. At this point in time I am convinced this gesture, this turn towards me, is enough.

I am still gulping air. "Here," I say.

I sit down on the grass next to her, lay my head on her belly. I listen for a life. Mine and who knows what other.

THE OTHER ONE DIED

That Saturday I was up early. I sat in front of the television watching George Jetson being dragged around by his overgrown Great Dane. Elroy, his son, was trying to get the dog to stop running.

"You coming today?" My dad walked into the family room holding a cup of coffee. He was wearing his Saturday morning clothes: baggy plaid pants, an old polo shirt with a penguin on the breast, and white deck shoes with lots of holes in them. My mother kept throwing these away, but he always dug them out of the trash. She didn't throw them in the outside trash cans, but in the bathroom where he would see them and save them. I continued eating cold pizza, leftovers from the night before.

"I thought we'd try Orange today." Every week we went to a flea market. Sometimes Orange, sometimes Santa Ana, or other places near where we lived in Southern California.

Then the phone rang and I knew it would be her. My mother was still in bed. She liked to sleep in Saturdays. We usually left the house around seven-thirty. My dad grabbed the phone off the wall near the television before it had a chance to ring twice.

"Feeling lucky?" he asked, "You got a thermos of coffee?" He hung up, satisfied.

"Ready, Cheeper?" He cuffed my ears. I was nine and looked seven. I turned off the TV and stuffed the rest of the pizza between two napkins. It was a thirty-minute ride to Orange; we'd be there before eight. "Get a move on, girl!" he said, and I scrambled to find a sweater.

Lilly lived a couple blocks away on Calle Camino. She told me once it meant "Street Street." As soon as we turned the corner, I could see her standing in front of her small house. Actually she leaned against the mailbox, one leg tucked up against her knee like a crane. Her right hand steadied herself on the mailbox and the other clutched a thin cane, like a divining rod. She often balanced like this; for her it was standing.

"Get the lead out!" she said as she folded herself into the front seat of the Volkswagon. "I've been waiting here for hours. We'll miss the bargains!" It had been less than five minutes since my dad talked with her on the phone. I was curled up in the little compartment in the very back of the tiny car. My mother called it the well. When I rode back there, she called me "the frog in the well."

"Ye gadz, pizza for breakfast!" She said this every week as if she didn't already know it was my favorite breakfast food.

"Hi, Lilly." I said this between mouthfuls.

"Still after some skates?" Lilly was cheerful in the morning. I nodded. She said, "Today's the day, I'll bet."

During the ride she and my father talked, but I could hardly hear what they were saying. From time to time Lilly dug into her macramé bag and pulled out a copy of *The Flea Market Trader* or some other book that would tell them the value of the stuff they had bought last week or were looking for this week. Lilly used to teach at the high school where my mother taught English, but she quit when her sickness got bad. Lilly and my mother were friends, too, but now she usually just visited with my father. My mother told me Lilly only had six months to live.

I sat in the back of the car and wondered why she wanted to buy things at flea markets if she only had six months to live. What would happen to it all after she died? I didn't think she had any children, or maybe she did, but they lived far away with their father. Today she had on a bright blue scarf that covered most of her head. I could still see a bald patch through the back where it was tied. It looked like my cat's belly after he had been scratching.

We got there early enough to get a parking spot near the gate. Some days we dropped Lilly off and then drove to find a parking space so she wouldn't have to walk too much. The flea markets were big, and she always insisted on walking every row. "What if there's a bargain there?" she said as she leaned against my father's arm and made it down the last aisle. "I'd hate to think of someone else getting it."

We bought admission tickets and my dad bought them coffee and me a donut. It was empty enough so I could wander around by myself and still find them easily. I liked to find out if there were any puppies or kittens there, and then I'd spend some time playing with them. I was looking for some skates, but good ones, not ones that were old and beat-up. I usually covered the whole place twice in the time it took them to see half of it.

My dad looked for old tools, golf balls and certain types of Coca-Cola trays. He knew just what kinds were old enough and rare enough to be worth something. One time he got one that said *Tome Coca-Cola* and that was worth a lot. It was Spanish.

Lilly combed through the stacks of plates and dishes. She knew which were worth a lot and which were fakes. She would lean against her cane and pick down with her other hand, and sometimes she'd look like a chicken picking in the dirt for seeds. Some days she and my dad would work as a team and pretend all kinds of things. Sometimes they would pretend they didn't know each other at all, and she would pick up a plate that was real expensive, and my dad would say, "That old thing, it isn't worth half of what they want." Then he'd laugh at her and turn away. Then she'd offer a lower price to the seller and sometimes she'd get it. This Saturday that I'm talking about they pretended they were husband and wife.

I saw them over at this big table of dishes. Lilly was starting to look through a stack of plates that had been taped together with masking tape. They were all different colors and patterns. She undid the tape, took the top one and turned it over to see the marking on the back. She kept looking through them, one by one, until she was about halfway through the pile. There were about twenty plates in that stack. Then this big puffy lady came over and grabbed what was left of the stack.

"You see the sticker, ten dollars for the stack. I had these taped together and now you've messed them all up!" She took the other plates from Lilly and tried to fix the tape around the pile. The sun was hot and the top plate was covered with little lines of sticky stuff like snail trailings. These were left by the tape.

"I just wanted to look through them to see if any of them matched the set I have," Lilly told the lady. She never let on that she was a collector. "I am trying to find one that matches because I broke one of my set and I am just sick about it." She said this with a really sweet voice, the kind you use when you are making fun of someone. People looked at her and the lady looked around, not sure what was going on. My dad came over and stood next to Lilly.

"What's the trouble, honey?" He held her arm and tried to look as innocent as he could. He isn't the innocent type.

"I want to find a plate to match my set and this lady won't let me look through this pile."

Sometimes people felt sorry for Lilly and let her buy things cheaper because they could see she was sick. But sometimes people didn't want to look at her or talk to her and were real mean. This lady behind the table didn't want Lilly around.

"No, ten dollars for the stack, and it's a bargain at that." The lady turned her back and I think she thought Lilly would go away. But Lilly really wanted to see the rest of those dishes. My dad approached from another angle.

"Excuse me, ma'am? I think there is one that matches my wife's set just there at the bottom. If you would be so kind as to let us look at it we'd be happy to pay ten dollars for these dishes." It wasn't the way my dad usually talked. It was funny to hear him call Lilly his wife. For a second I wondered what she would be like as my mother, but then I remembered she was going to die. Also, I liked my mother.

"Listen, mister, I told you the plates are a package deal. Ten dollars for the stack." She was angry because we had been standing in front of her table for a while and no one else could see her stuff. Plus I think she didn't like us and knew we didn't like her. She stared right at Lilly and then took the plates and set them just out of Lilly's reach.

"We'll take those plates, thank you very much." Lilly had dropped her sweet candy voice. She dug in her purse and handed over a ten dollar bill. I had never seen Lilly pay more than five dollars for anything. Other people were watching, too. My dad looked a little surprised. He went to pick up the plates. I'll bet he was wondering how he was going to drag them around the rest of the flea market. Sometimes the sellers let you store stuff with them while you walk around, but this lady wasn't going to be one of those.

Lilly called to me and asked me to hold her cane. She shuffled over and picked up the stack of plates and it looked like she was going to fall forward with the weight of them. She scooped them into her arms and slowly took a step back away from the table. The lady was watching her, so was everyone else. She moved slow, and you could tell something was going to happen from the look in her eyes.

She looked up at the lady and then down at the plates. Then she dropped them — the whole stack — on the black asphalt. About half of them shattered and some of them cracked. One rolled away unhurt out into the middle of the aisle. My dad started to laugh. So did Lilly. I watched the lady, who got really red in her face.

Lilly said, "Well, there was one that matched in that stack." That made my dad laugh harder, and Lilly grabbed her cane from me and put her arm through his. They walked away, slowly, laughing. Other people laughed, too. I went to save the plate that didn't break. The lady called after us, "Come back here and clean this up!"

Lilly slept in the car on the way home. She usually did. I sat in the back seat and rolled my new skates against the opposite window. The leather of the shoe part was clean, but the wheels were cheap. My dad said he'd change the wheels for me. There was a box of golf balls in the well that rocked when the car went around corners and sounded a bit like the rocks on the beach when the waves rolled over them. I was tired, too.

It was still before noon when we got home. There was a note on the refrigerator from my mom, "At the beach, join me?" She always put a smiley face on her notes. I went to change into my bathing suit.

My dad didn't like the beach so much. He didn't like the sand and how it got everywhere. After we ate some lunch I rode my bike to the beach. He went out to play golf. Later that night all three of us went to the movies. I can't remember what we saw.

Lilly didn't die that year. My dad did. One day he just died, playing golf, and we never got to say good-bye or anything. It didn't seem fair.

Lilly got better, in fact, and now she walks without a cane or anything. I don't see her much because she moved further away, but sometimes she calls and asks me if I want her to keep an eye out for something special at the flea market. For my birthday she bought me a great table. It's made of sticks and shaped like an elephant. I think she probably got it at the flea market. I don't know about my dad and Lilly. I liked her, though.

THE GETTING OF KNOWLEDGE

I suppose it depends on what you know already — I mean, how much there is for you to learn in college. Coming out of high school, I knew nothing.

The first night in my dorm room underscored this knowing of nothing. (You know, underscore, like when you take those yellow and blue highlighter pens and scratch under anything that sounds vaguely conclusive?) I was putting away my new college wardrobe (bought with my earnings from waitressing at Howard Johnson's); hanging the new London Fog next to the three sensible skirts, setting my brown loafers on the floor of the tiny cupboard which I supposed was meant to be a closet. Four of us were to live in two boxed-in rooms; a sleeping compartment as small as a bathroom with two sets of bunk beds tucked next to each other — less than a foot between them — and a study with four cubicled desks and a wire-framed chair behind each.

"I can't believe what a good lover Ron is," Alexis says this to Jules and Frances, who know each other already from freshman year. "I come almost every time, without even trying." Jules smiles and nods her head. I continue to stack the $168.58 worth of fat, heavy textbooks on the foot-long shelf which is somehow supposed to hold all of them. These I have just purchased after waiting through three-hour lines at the university bookstore. Frances stands in front of a mirror and runs her fingers through the length of her blonde bob. She is nearly six feet tall and wears skin-tight jeans and a pale-pink sweatshirt.

"Well, I continued to see Jimmy all summer. And quite simply," she stops with her voice high in the air and turns on her flat pink pumps to face Jules and Frances. "Quite simply," she repeats, "we fucked our brains out." With this she laughs and drops into Jules' lap throwing her head over Jules' left shoulder and placing a well-manicured right hand just above the neckline of her sweatshirt. They laugh.

Frances tells about her affair with her cousin at their beach house: sand and salt and all the ingredients I would imagine go into such a summer romance. I think of Hojo's and how all summer I dated a guy who worked in the kitchen and we made out in his Chevy Luv truck behind the high school. We did, that is, until we got busted by the cops. For what? Curfew or something. I was so busy pulling up my bra and down my blouse I can't remember what the cop said. But anyway, I'm thinking of all this and how me and Henry never went beyond third base — maybe to third and a half — and I've never even had an orgasm and suddenly I want to go home and continue waitressing at Hojo's where we didn't talk about sex, not much, and never about orgasms.

But Frances has turned to me and asked, "Ellen, what's your sex life like?" Just like that, as if it had a life of its own.

I look up from my desk and say politely, "Excuse me? I wasn't listening to your conversation."

How this can be true in a ten-by-ten room with four of us in it is beyond me and them, too, I expect. But to cover myself I say, "I'm bushed. What time's breakfast in the morning?"

Without waiting for an answer I walk past them, up the hall and into the communal bathroom where I sit on the toilet and vow to fuck someone before the end of the first semester.

An orgasm?

If I'm lucky.

I learned a lot that first year. Alexis broke up with Ron, Frances started to date a football player, and Jules and Jimmy exchanged a series of phone calls that interrupted our sleep nearly every night. Frances and her football player slept in a corner of our study room in a nest she concocted from blankets and an old mattress she retrieved from the basement of the dorm. Every night I listened to them doing it, mostly just his deep moaning after five or ten minutes of muffled thrashing, and every morning I stepped lightly over the two lumps of their bodies as I made my way to breakfast.

I changed my major from poli sci to English after a run in with the Head of Department, a short, nervous man with a blanket of dandruff on the shoulders of his dark, shiny suits. After class one day near the end of term we started talking about my career. He climbed up on a bench so he towered two feet above me.

"Germs," he said in explanation to the air above my head. "Everywhere. Up here I'll miss yours and you mine."

The tick in the left side of his face started doing its calisthenics. I craned my head back and told him I worked nights and weekends waiting tables and that I couldn't afford to take the internship he'd found me, in a law firm, without any pay.

"God," he said, flipping the long side of his hair across the bald egg of his head, "Waitressing. *Waitressing*." I walked slowly backwards as he began to rave about "getting somewhere in life." His hands flew and the hair that he had placed so carefully over his head slipped from position and stuck out stiffly at a right angle from his ear like a shelf or antenna. I was all for getting somewhere in life, but first I had to pay tuition.

That night I went out with a boy from my classics class. Neither of us had a car and so we walked in the rain, eating pizza, reciting lines from Shakespeare and later wound up having sex in one of the soundproof music rooms in the library. We slept all night there. It was okay. No orgasm but I think I came close.

English was the ticket. No more clunky and expensive textbooks. I could buy my books at secondhand stores and take the slim novels everywhere. I could look suave and sophisticated propped behind a copy of Plato's *Dialogues*, or sit in a café in front of a steamy mug of mud-colored coffee or a juice glass of cheap red wine reading romantic poetry. One night I cut the front of my shoulder length hair to half-inch long and dyed the rest red. I dumped the guy from classics. I loved my professors. Especially the Drs. Halloway.

Jay Halloway and his wife Marge Halloway had offices across the hall from each other in the small damp building that housed the English department. Jay was tall with sandy hair and wore turtlenecks, jeans and sports jackets with leather elbow patches. In his classes — Black Writers of the Harlem Renaissance, The Literature of the American Dream, Beat Poets — we talked politics and culture, listened to jazz and blues on his portable stereo, and saw slides of protests and civil rights marches. With Marge — a lanky, dark-haired woman with deep blue eyes — I learned about feminism. We studied Virginia Woolf, Willa Cather, the early work of Alice Walker. Collectively we became enraged and enlightened. I stopped wearing skirts, bought jeans and an entire wardrobe (in black) from the Goodwill. I moved out of the dorm, lost track of Alexis, Jules and Frances, and into a cooperative where I learned to smoke pot and cook stir-fry vegetables.

But this story isn't about my fashion development, or my culinary skills, but my getting of knowledge. And so back to the Halloways. Over those four years — that chunk of time they call the very best of life — I grew to worship Marge and Jay and their marriage. They had two toddlers, girls, and Jay took them Mondays and Tuesdays and Marge took them Thursdays and Fridays. I watched them on Wednesdays. Their wood-burning stove kept the place warm while I studied. I planned graduate school, a man like Jay and a life like theirs. Occasionally I had boyfriends (and orgasms, I was pleased to discover) and then it was time to graduate.

The English department's annual end-of-the-year bash was held at the Halloways'. There were flagons of red wine, a keg in the bathtub, the Stones on the stereo. Triscuits, brie and raw vegetables were scattered throughout the downstairs in small clay bowls. Though it was June, there was still a chill in the air and the wood stove coughed and groaned throughout the evening. I drank a lot and wove myself around the packed living room, already morose with nostalgia.

Marge leaned up against the sink in the kitchen talking with a group of freshmen girls about the Bloomsbury crowd, her dissertation topic. I recognized my earlier self in them; they hung on her words, noted her gestures, caught each shred of information carefully in the loose netting of their brains.

I tried to leave the kitchen, but facing the oncoming traffic, I suddenly felt faint and nauseous. Ducking left into the pantry, I slipped open the basement door. I thought it might be cooler there and I feared losing the cheap wine and the dozens of black olives that seemed to bob up and down in my stomach like so many buoys on a rough sea.

At the top of the stairs, I touched the light switch just as I heard the muffled sound of what could only be body against body. But the sound reached my ears too late and the message from brain to finger had already been activated. A single hanging bulb lit up the musty and damp basement; I saw the creamy white ass of Jay Halloway on its upswing, a dark birthmark the size of a quarter and the shape of Africa like a target taunting me from in the middle of his tight left cheek.

"Excuse me," I said and turned around, but not before I heard a familiar voice.

"Hi, Ellen."

It was the voice of Alexis, the bimbo roommate from freshman year. I hadn't seen her for ages, had almost forgotten about her. I said "Hi, Alexis" then flipped the light switch off, walked back up stairs and out the front door.

I kept in touch with the Halloways, wrote them from graduate school, acknowledged them in the front of my dissertation. I wrote on sexual imagery in the novels of the American dream. At the time it seemed like what I needed to know.

BLUEPRINTS FOR MODERN LIVING

This period is only a historical accident.
— Isabel Allende

The Earth's Rotation

I wake feeling as though I am in the belly of a giant whale. I lie still in my bed, braced for a toss and a tumble, unsure. The rolling stops and I sit up on my elbows, queasy from seasickness, or not enough sleep. The house groans, starts rumbling, and I realize: another earthquake.

Watching the lights sway, I think about standing under a door frame, but instead my gaze is drawn to a print, framed and under glass, directly above my pillow. I've considered moving it, imagining it crashing upon me in the midst of The Big One. The day after an earthquake the papers are splashed with predictions: "Scientists Say Big Quake Overdue" or, depending on the paper, "Disaster Imminent!" I gave up reading those articles and I've never read Jeanne Dixon's yearly forecasts in the *Enquirer*. It's not that I think they're a sham, or hokey, or even scientifically unsound. It's just that at this point in my life I'll gladly trade surety for a sense of possibility, even if that possibility spells disaster.

The print does not fall, yet I imagine my obituary: "The deceased survived by . . ." Who? Whom am I survived by? We all survive because we all survive — it's not poetic, I know. But given that when we all go — whether it's because of that black hole spreading across the ozone or because our man in D.C. decides to show who's boss — we'll all go together. Individual deaths aren't of interest anymore, they hardly make the news. The day of this earthquake we all survive, every last one of us mad enough to live on this lovable fault we call home.

The neighborhood dogs begin their morning *a cappella* concert. I do not go outside. I do not start to bottle water. I do not switch off the gas. No, I turn on the television and learn I — and all of us — have lived through a medium-sized tremor, four-something on Mr. Richter's scale. I expect we'll watch the world's grand finale on "Good Morning America." Will Bryant Gumbel sign off for us all? A few aftershocks murmur under my bare feet like the faint waves of pleasure after orgasm. I climb back into my still-toasty bed and fall back asleep. And the phone rings.

"You all right?" It is my mother calling from Florida. "Honey?"

"I'm fine. It was just a small one."

She calls every time there's an earthquake, incredulous that I live in California, which she is sure will soon join Hawaii in the Pacific Ocean. I, however, am appalled that she lives in Florida, where each year she gets friendly with a hurricane and for weeks calls it by name. "Flora is still on her way," she assures me as if Flora was dropping in for a cup of tea. She lives through hurricanes. My sister in Oregon lives through ice storms. I live through earthquakes. We all make our choices, I suppose, based on what we can endure. Somehow I prefer my disaster to come from below, from the shifting of the world's crusty plates; Ma Kettle's indigestion.

"I've got to go to work, Mom." I lie. However, she readily agrees to get off the phone. Long distance is a modern extravagance she has never fully accepted. I have seen her phone bill, each long distance entry is noted — after the number and price is a word, the cause for the call. Last time I visited I watched her make these markings. "Birthday" she wrote under a call to my sister in Oregon. "Death" she scratched over a Michigan entry. I can imagine her penciling in the word "Earthquake" alongside my Berkeley, California number.

The Day's Rotation

Hardly anyone talks about the earthquake for the rest of the day. It's Saturday and I meet my friend Lenny at a café because we've decided to go to a protest together. Sometimes I read about New York where people of our age (that age right before thirty when all is not possible nor even probable anymore) meet at gallery openings or rock clubs and put more up their noses in a half hour than Lenny and I make in a day. In Berkeley we meet at bookstores or protests, or over a cappuccino in one of the many cafés near the university. Walking between the divided lots of people on historic Telegraph Avenue — the street people, flanked by dogs, army packs and shopping bags, and the young, optimistic, selectively-sighted university students dressed in bright colors harsh against the gray and luminous sky — we slip invisibly into anonymity. Here, next to the polluted San Francisco Bay, guarded by the picture-perfect Golden Gate Bridge, we live lives undocumented by the media. Somewhere between yuppies and hippies we latent members of the baby boom drive around the potholed, palm-tree-lined streets of California in Valiants and old Volvos trying, unsuccessfully and without validation, to place our lives into historical context.

Lenny and I work at a newspaper, a lefty sort of newspaper, and we set type which is a romantic way of saying that we sit in front of computer terminals and get paid twice as much as secretaries for essentially the same work. Lenny is very good at it, which means he understands exactly how the machine unravels the commands we punch in. I don't understand the machine and when faced with a problem usually start pressing buttons indiscriminately in the hopes of controlling what I sense is an arbitrary electronic process. About once a week I lose entire stories as a result of my impatience with computer logic — and where they go I've no idea. I'll be working along, talking with Lenny about the Faulkner book he's been reading, or about my girlfriend, or about his marriage breaking up, and then while reaching for my coffee I'll brush the keyboard and the whole thing vanishes. Poof! It has to do with "appending" and "replacing" and I try to keep very concrete pictures in my head of old-fashioned file cabinets so as to do the right one at the right time. But as I say, the machine usually wins and eats the story just as I've finished typing it in. It's usually something long and boring about parking, or city politics, or a letter to the editor about dog shit on our streets, and then I have to gear up to start all over, or take a coffee break. I'm not a good typesetter but it's a union shop and they'd have a hard time getting rid of me. Sometimes that's the irony of leftist organizing: If I was stuck with me as a typesetter I'd think twice about unions.

Lenny is sitting at the café drinking black coffee out of a

pint-sized styrofoam cup and eating a dry bagel. He's been dieting ever since his wife left him. Actually, she didn't leave him, she said she needed some space and then bought it. They got married six years ago after knowing each other for three months, a leap of faith in the best of times but in those days it must have been fueled by fervent and illogical hope. Marriage and commitment have gained popularity over the last few years, but Lenny got married at a time when anything more than living together seemed like a throwback to the fifties. He believes in marriage, in love, and in some ways, justice. Coupled with his devotion to good books, this is what makes Lenny interesting to me. I — who at twelve could not fathom what was described to me as the Holocaust and who in my early twenties truly believed the ERA would pass, and who at twenty-eight could not begin to understand the minds who not only thought up such a plan as Star Wars, but had the audacity to start building space shields — I found myself rooting for Lenny's marriage with the zeal of a high school cheerleader. It's an interesting alliance, Lenny and I, one my girlfriend and his wife — possibly ex-wife — are just beginning to understand. Friendship between a straight man and a lesbian is rare, even in Berkeley.

"Hey, skinny," I say, pulling up a chair and setting my salmon covered bagel on the coffee-stained table. Lenny sits hunched over the morning newspaper, his well worn jean jacket on the chair beside him, his white, button-down shirt tucked into a pair of deep blue — new, I suppose — Levi 501s. Lenny's hair looks as if it houses a family of mice. Falling well below his ears, his brown, fine curls often cover his eyes. Sometimes when he typesets he'll take one hand and brush the hair from his forehead, sometimes when it isn't there. He's still a faster typist than me, even with that one hand waving about.

"Hey," Lenny says, looking up.

"What's news?" I ask.

The front page of the paper is covered with photographs, a frame-by-frame account of a train in the act of running over an anti-war protester. Against my intentions I find myself scrutinizing the photos, looking for an expression on the engineer's face that will explain something to me, looking for a sign that would signify why god would allow another atrocity. All I see is a child, holding his head with both hands as his stepfather loses both legs, and a bride of eight days rushing to her husband's side trying to hold blood within her husband's body with only the torn hem of her skirt.

"Did you feel the earthquake?" I ask, tearing my eyes away from the paper. I feel slightly nauseous thinking about the man's foot, severed and autonomous lying on the railroad tracks, discarded and limp like a day-old newspaper. I move the lox across the table.

"I slept right though it," he says through a bite of his bagel. We sit there for a moment, Lenny chewing, me thinking about him sleeping through the quake. He grew up in California, in one of those cities clustered around Los Angeles that all seem the same to me, in a home not unlike mine, though mine sat in a similar suburb in Michigan. Our parents are middle-class, Christian, Republican. They watched us grow up safely in the chasm between the sixties and drugs and the eighties and money. Coming of age in the seventies was like being in that middle part of the tennis court my father calls "no man's land"; too far forward to catch balls at the baseline, too far back to play the net. I watched my older sister smoke pot in the garage, protest Vietnam on television, live with a succession of men, arrange at least two abortions and survive a number of "bad trips." Is this what I missed by being born too late? Now, she is married to a school-teacher and is raising two sons in a small city in Oregon. On weekends she and Rick, now her husband after eight years of being her "man," pile the kids into an old station wagon and pull a small egg-shaped trailer to the country where they fish and, when the kids fall asleep, smoke tightly rolled joints. I think this is what Lenny had expected for himself and his bride, Kate. But Kate decided to go into computers, started making big money and thus: her own condo overlooking the bay, complete with a creamy leather couch and pink Levolors. Lenny lives in their old place, a rented cottage in a quirky neighborhood below the university. He kept their record collection. Kate uprooted the herb garden and took it, potted, to her condo. "Can't live without my basil," she said. Lenny now calls her The Pesto Queen.

There is not much to say about the morning's news.

"How's Maggie?" Lenny says, and I say "Fine" even though there's a lot I could say. There is a way being friends with Lenny has got built-in safety catches, for both of us. It's not going to be complicated by matters of love or lust, and the way that we don't know the realities of each others' lives keeps everything so safe.

Sometimes, guiltily, I feel like I'm looking at Lenny through "Wild Kingdom" glasses, like he's a rare bird and I'm documenting his mating patterns.

"Kate's seeing José," he adds.

"Seeing, or *seeing?*"

"Sleeping with."

"That explains the Spanish language course," I say and laugh and immediately regret it.

"Thanks," he says into his coffee.

I try to redeem myself. "She's a jerk."

He smiles. He's got these doe-like eyes, moist and soft and his right hand gracefully flutters across his forehead sweeping the hair from his head. I'm forgiven. I vow not to be so coarse. I want people like Lenny in my life.

"Let's go," he says.

I wrap my bagel in a paper napkin and stick it in the pocket of my tattered leather jacket. We are going to the train tracks where the man was run over.

At the Edge of the Tide

Inland, the windless country is dry and hot. We leave our jackets in my old red Valiant and join the crowds of people walking towards the weapons station. I bought the Valiant from my sister when she left for college years ago, for the fair and reasonable sum of five hundred dollars. In high school and later in college, kids laughed at my red beast; such a tank, such an old folks' car, they'd say. Over the past few years — thanks to the union — I've given her a new paint job, reupholstered her seats, cleaned up her original engine. Now I am offered substantial amounts of money for her by the same people who laughed me out of the high school parking lot. "Wanna sell?" they'll ask me from their Honda civics. "Fat chance," I spit back, my voice betraying some bitterness. Besides, I had my first girl in the back seat, Carrie Sue Thomas, after the Homecoming football game senior year. My mother recently reported that Carrie Sue is married and selling real estate in St. Paul.

There are hundreds going to protest: old, young, families carrying picnics, dogs on and off leashes. As we approach the site, we are accosted by all forms of fliers thrust at us like the arms of turnstiles at the grocery store, brightly colored sheets of paper covered by type so dense they're less inviting than a Republican fundraiser. Each splinter of every communist or socialist group tries to pass its party line to the already-converted masses as if the protest was a revival meeting and they are fighting for our lost souls. Both Lenny and I keep our hands deep in our pockets and shake our heads at every invitation. I spot a woman I know who works at a large multinational. She is wearing a long black wig and passing out leaflets for the Marxist-Leninists. I'm sure she doesn't want to be recognized and I'm glad I can slip by her flailing arms without notice.

A stage is set up near the train tracks, hay has been spread on the dirt and the lines for the Porta-Johns are already twenty deep. From this small spot on the dry California landscape our military ships guns and missiles to Nicaragua, the Persian Gulf, and who knows where else? First they — and when I say "they" I can only think of faceless, clean-shaven young men, both black and white (indistinguishable in their mottled army fatigues), sweat dripping from their temples under our warm winter sun — they load them onto trains, such as the train that ran over the now-legless man. The weapons are driven to the sea and make their way to the Pacific. Slipping silently under the Golden Gate Bridge, the weapons — the guns and missiles and whatever else is packed in those crates marked boldly for the world to see — become our offering to the peoples of this planet.

Lenny is unusually silent. He sits down between the Gray Panthers and the Vietnam vets. I cannot think of a more perfect place to sit, between inspiration and hope. The vets stand at attention: Mirrored sunglasses cover emotion. Worn jeans poke out from beneath flak jackets or ribboned and bejeweled military coats. Pony-tails snake down the backs of two men holding the ends of a purple and gold fringed banner: "Vietnam Veterans Opposed to U.S. Militarism." Against all intellect, my heart swells. For a moment I feel like an unmarried gal in the streets of New York on V-Day. I want to jump up and kiss the tall, lanky stranger on my left, hungry for that bravery to rub off upon my lips. Yet I can't help but think of them as both brave and foolish as if they have taken a hairpin turn on Highway 1 on a rainy and wet, black winter's night — and come out laughing, bleary-eyed, tears tracking the crevices of their cheeks.

The gray-haired woman to my right looks not unlike my mother, save for a "U.S. Out of Central America" button pinned to the collar of her polyester shell. She is passing fried chicken to her friends, pouring coffee from a red thermos. Lenny and I have brought a pint of mineral water and two Hershey bars. I imagine her frying that chicken early in the morning, wrapping it in Saran Wrap and placing each piece in a Tupperware box, like any woman preparing for a picnic, a car trip — a protest? The man I think is her husband clasps a clipboard to his chest, a petition that he offers me and that I sign without reading. I am convinced that whatever this couple believes in, I must believe in, too. I smile and hand the clipboard back to him. "Thanks," I say and the woman offers me a serene smile between sips of coffee. The domesticity of the scene has not escaped Lenny's notice. He takes the clipboard and signs his name to the list of believers, and I suspect both of us want to ask the same questions: How did you get this far together? How do you keep believing?

Riding Out the Current

Lenny is weeping, quietly, on the passenger's side of the Valiant on the way back from the protest. The protest was successful, I suppose, in numerical terms. And Joan Baez sang the Lord's Prayer and Jesse Jackson got us to stand, hands clasped and raised against the glaring sun. I'm driving and talking about time. I am interested in the way people visualize life on those picture screens in our heads. And I'm nervous about Lenny crying.

"In my mind life looks like a series of building blocks, only there are turns at certain points," I try to explain. I trace a path along the inside of the dirty windshield and Lenny wipes his eyes and looks at the snakelike diagram.

"Here's birth," I point to the near end of the snake. "Then there's this curve around to here, that's about ten years old, and then there's this long stretch here that reaches to thirty." I glance at Lenny and I see that he's stopped crying and has pulled his hair down over his brow so I can hardly see his eyes. I'm sure he doesn't want me to see him cry, and I'm not sure I want to anyway. "I'm just at this turn, here, and then I slide over the hill and down to forty. How does a life look in your mind?"

I've always been interested in how people organize concepts in their heads. I have another diagram in my head for the twenty-four hours of the day which has curves and twists similar to the life-snake. I have a blimp-like picture in my mind for the seven days of the weeks, and a strange "D" pattern for the year which inexplicably gives extra space to the summer months. Maggie, my girlfriend, says she has no organizing patterns for time, and watching her live, I am apt to believe her. With the turn of thirty before me, I am more interested than ever in these mental blueprints.

Lenny doesn't answer me. Instead he starts to cry again, full force.

"Don't cry," I say foolishly and try to merge with oncoming traffic while watching Lenny's thin chest heave and rock. "Everything will work out." This is something I hear on bad TV movies and I am somewhat shocked to hear myself say it. I've never seen Lenny cry like this before — in fact, never seen a man cry like this ever. Crying women sound like small captured animals, raspy with sharp noises coming from somewhere in the back of their throats. Lenny sounds like a harpooned whale; bursts of long and low pitched sound come up from his belly. He's crying harder and louder, and I am frantic trying to figure out what to do, what to say, how to stay within the white lines of the freeway and the cool corridors of our friendship.

Pulling off at the first exit, I drive into the parking lot of a giant Safeway. I park the Valiant alongside a recycling trailer and Lenny doubles over his knees. His head touches the dash. Slowly, I slide over the front seat and place one hand across Lenny's wide back. His body rises and falls as he tries to regain his breath. My touch is light, but I can feel warmth coming through his shirt.

"Lenny?" I ask. "Hey, Lenny?"

His back falls one more time and he straightens up in the car. My hand is pinned between him and the seat. And then I see his face, twisted and tight, and his red, puffy eyes, and I begin to cry. And I am crying for Lenny because his wife isn't going to come back to him, and I believe even if she did he wouldn't want her. And I'm crying because losing two legs is both too much and too little in this war we are waging against the world. And I'm crying because I'm about to turn that corner in my mind and slide over thirty and I have no career, no babies, no husband, no picket fence. And now Lenny is holding me, and I him, and though I haven't held a man since 1979 when my father and I went camping and he turned his ankle and I had to carry him through the forest, this holding seems as natural as apple pie and ice cream. Twice the size of Maggie, Lenny rests against my chest with the weight of a wall of water. Both of us are crying.

Shoring Up

I left Lenny at a café where he was meeting a friend. There was something new between us, a sadness and a hope, as if we had jointly lived through a crisis or disaster, though whatever happened to each of us that day happened quite separately as well as together. I drove to Maggie's house where she was busy at the stove concocting a kind of goulash. I ate heartily, mounds of potatoes and carrots, sopping up the brown gravy with huge hunks of sour bread. After dinner I planned my own birthday party, making long lists of guests and supplies. I don't want to be alone when I turn that corner.

That night there was another earthquake, smaller than the one that morning. They called it an aftershock. I wondered if Lenny slept through that one, too.

THINGS YOU CAN NEVER KNOW

I was holding up a black wool dress, *circa* 1940, with a low neckline and bugle bead trim on the sleeves and bodice. The price was right — four-fifty — and there was a chance I could fit into it, but — pun intended — a slim one.

"Very *bee*-ut-i-ful," the male voice came from behind me. The accent was strong, not unusual in the Mission district.

I turned, expecting I-don't-know-what: my lips tightly pressed together, a no-nonsense stance. But I'll admit: I'm the kind of feminist who will walk past a site of jeering construction workers with all intentions of telling them off, yet somehow end up flashing a coy smile. At forty, my smile is one of my best-preserved assets.

"A very *bee*-ut-i-ful dress," he said. "I will buy it for you and you will wear it on our date."

Bee-ut-i-ful, indeed. Sharp cheekbones, almost Indian, smooth brown skin, coal black hair, ragged over the ears and collar. Not young, mid-thirties. Nevertheless, with proper grooming he could be a *GQ* man. But the flared jeans and a faded black Iron Maiden t-shirt gave him away as a recent arrival. Somewhat embarrassed by his handsomeness, I studied the dress. The bust: ample. The waist? Possible.

"No shopping?" he questioned, staring openly at my t-shirt.

I had come from the pro-choice rally at the Federal Building. My shirt sported a red circle with a slash printed over a coat hanger.

"No, it's about abortion. They use coat hangers — like these —" I shook the one with the dress, "for illegal abortions. Right now there's a threat to the law —" I started rattling off my spiel as if I were canvassing door to door.

"You must talk slow," he said. "And explain to me when we are drinking coffee."

That was six weeks ago. A Sunday. We had coffee at the Clarion, my choice, and later dinner at a tiny Mexican restaurant where, during the week, Miguel washes dishes. That night at my apartment, after describing to me San Salvador (and before you get the idea I was wooed by a refugee revolutionary: He came to this country to learn to fly planes and make money), I tried to explain the politics of pro-choice.

"Sad," he said and shook his head. "Abortions no good. Not good for God." His face was drawn and long, and against all better judgment, I reached across the couch and touched his silky hair. He brightened, we kissed, and later, the rest. Still later I tried on the dress — it fit, tight — and he told me I looked like a Hollywood movie star.

In 1970, when I was a senior in college, I waitressed at Sambo's to pay my tuition. Three weeknights, ten to two, and Saturday night until four a.m., I paced the twenty feet of counter space, refilled endless cups of coffee for the regulars, and delivered pie and hot fudge sundaes to parades of pot heads. All this dressed in a ridiculous outfit: a peasant blouse of fake patchwork and an orange micro-mini skirt. I also wore the requisite ruffled bloomers and plastic name tag: Kate — short for Katherine. And against restaurant policy (wedding or engagement rings only) I wore a small brass peace symbol on a thin strand of leather tied around my neck. When it was slow I read paperbacks of Dostoevski and Marx, thwarted advances from the cooks, and made small talk with various regulars who, if courted, might leave a dollar tip on a three-hour cup of coffee.

For a while my boyfriend, Mike, came to the restaurant during my shift and parked himself at the end of my counter. Fair, long-haired and tie-dyed, he was looking for debate on the war, and sometimes the well-shorn, khaki-clad boys from the nearby military base took him on. After a few more-than-heated discussions, the skinny night manager ushered me into the cold freezer, and instructed me to leave my entourage at home, or lose my job. So Mike bowed out of Sambo's.

That's when I met Ole. The first few times I saw him I hardly got past the uniform, but one night, pouring a refill, I looked past his military garb into a face I couldn't look away from: deep blue eyes, tanned Nordic skin, pale hair as soft as a duck's underbelly. He was charming and polite, from Michigan, and he told me he enlisted in the service for the free doctor's education. He left a dollar on a cup of coffee.

Ole knew I was against the war, the military, and just about everything else at that time, and I knew he was being trained to kill, if not also to clean up afterwards. If it wasn't young love, it was certainly lust: My heart fired its own artillery when I saw him stride through the double glass doors and swivel his lovely khaki-clad ass onto a bright orange stool. One night we took a hotel room, and I explained to Mike I had to work the entire graveyard shift, ten to six. For three weeks I worked graveyard with Ole, and then he was shipped out. A month later he sent me a letter, at the restaurant, postmarked in South Carolina. If he sent more, I never knew. I was fired a few weeks later.

Even through the full peasant blouse, I was starting to show.

My daughter, now twenty, looks like a female version of a 1970s Mike. She's wearing a tie-dyed t-shirt with old jeans, and her blonde hair is long, tangled and twisted every which way. She's also wearing boxing gloves and dancing about in front of the mirror in my bedroom. I'm lying crosswise on my bed, flipping through the latest copy of *Cosmopolitan* magazine. The lead story is about "Changing Men." Impulsively, and not without a dash of blind hope, I snatched it at the check-out counter.

"Shadow boxing," Maxine explains, between swats at the mirror, "develops reflexes . . . good exercise . . . and aerobic endurance."

"Uh-huh," I say, despondently. The article is not about how to *change* men, but about how men are *changing*.

Boxing is Maxine's newest craze, following speedskating (too dangerous on the crowded Berkeley streets) and surfing (winter squelched that one) and half a dozen other athletic fads, including a one-day stint of sky diving.

"Knock-out!" Maxine lunges and punches, then steps back holding hands clasped above her head. "Champion!" She falls across the bed beside me.

"So Henry didn't go with you to the abortion rally," she says. Before boxing, we were discussing my recent problems with Henry, my boyfriend of the last five years.

"And now you're not talking?" she adds. "That's a bit extreme. That's not even like you, Mom."

Over the past several years my daughter has somehow become my romantic confidante. She's a junior at UC Berkeley, just across the bay, and she calls every few days to keep me posted on the who's-who of her sex life and what's-what of her future. I've learned to offer advice only when asked — rarely — and to take three deep breaths before letting any "mother-type judgments" — as Max calls them — slip out.

It was shocking at first, the shift away from mother, but I slowly opened up my personal life for commentary as well. And now this person I mothered for twenty years, monitoring her world of boys and sex and self-esteem, has become my friend. She's smart and perceptive, with a unique first-hand view of the last twenty years of my life, and — usually — she's surprisingly unprejudiced when giving advice. She's also quite different than I am, a lot more like Mike, certain and confident. Perhaps the summers spent with him in Vermont had great influence.

"I'm still talking to him," I tell her. "I'm just being, you know —"

"Unavailable emotionally," she says and turns towards me. Where does she gets this stuff? "You should tell him what's the matter," she says. "Talk to him. Otherwise nothing's going to change."

This is sound advice, I know, but Maxine has an angle. She likes this steady man in my life, thinks it would be good if I remarried. "Besides I wanted to ask you two to dinner Sunday. It's time you met Nadi." Nadi is Maxine's most recent beau, a Pakistani and Maxine's anti-Israeli comrade.

"Don't count on Henry for anything on Sundays. These days Sundays are reserved for football with the boys."

"*After* the game," she says, with some exasperation and rolls off the bed. "Besides it's not like Henry's a *jock*." To my daughter the radical, just as it was for me twenty years ago, being a jock is the worst; it somehow epitomizes the most base qualities of masculinity. "And he's only into football lately because the 'Niners are winning. *Everybody's* into football now. Ice cream?"

"Not for me," I say. She punches her way up the hall to the kitchen.

My Henry works in the next carrell over from me at the community law office, takes tenants' rights cases for low pay and sometimes fights both landlords and city hall simultaneously. Most of his clients are immigrants who are too scared of being turned over to immigration to fight the slum lords who are continually raising their rents. Henry is slender and sensitive and rarely leaves home without a wool muffler wrapped around his waist and tucked beneath his shirt and Levi's: His grandmother once told him that colds enter through the kidneys and he reveres her wisdom. In so many words: Henry is certainly no jock. But it's easier to put blame on Henry than the entire San Francisco football team, or even myself. Because if the 'Niners hadn't been winning, he wouldn't have been watching the game and he would have been at that abortion rally with me. We would have stopped at El Toro on the way home, picked up burritos and pineapple juice, tuned in "Sixty Minutes," and afterwards made love.

I would not have been shopping at Thriftown.

I would never have met Miguel.

Miguel comes over in the late afternoons, for coffee and Mexican biscuits, on his way to the restaurant. Often we make love, with great urgency and passion, before he slips into the foggy night air. He begs to come back after work, but so far I have staved him off with lies about my visiting daughter and/or early morning appointments. I've known him for five weeks now. He wants to marry me.

"Not for green card only," he says shaking his head from side to side.

He is sitting at the breakfast bar. The thin white t-shirt against his dark skin has gone a shade of light brown, like a translucent wrap over a piece of coffee taffy. Two browned hands, smooth despite the long hours immersed in soap suds, toy with a nerf football. It's Henry's football.

"Because of love," he says and smiles. I roll my eyes heavenwards and turning to the sink, begin to rinse our coffee mugs.

"Things aren't so simple," I say over the running water.

"Why not, simple?"

"They just aren't."

"Sunday you eat with my aunt and brother," he says. "Then next week I meet your Maxine. Then we get married."

I'm wondering when he and Henry are going to meet, can't imagine the introduction. Is there a masculine version of mistress? And does it apply to nonmarrieds?

Miguel is behind me now, nibbling on my ear. "We get married in the park?" He laughs. Last Sunday we saw two gay men getting married in Dolores Park. Miguel was transfixed by the open display of affection. He was also taken by the irreverence of an outdoor wedding.

His tongue retreats from my ear and his head cocks to one side. We both hear sirens, some distance away. Yesterday when it was time for him to go to work, there was a policemen on my street giving parking tickets. But Miguel, without papers or a visa, was immediately frightened, the blood drained from his face leaving him an eerie beige. He stayed inside until the cop left, a delay that made him late for work.

Now, the sounds of the sirens outside grow louder and I see that same fear in his otherwise relaxed and beautiful face. My heart pinches to see him so afraid of a fire truck.

"I'll marry you," I say without thinking, a response to a signal from my heart. "But just for immigration. Only for papers."

Miguel shuts his eyes, puts both hands over his heart, then drops to one knee before me on the kitchen floor. Kisses trail up my left leg.

"Really, Miguel. Just to make you legal."

"*Mi esposa*," he says, rising, nipping at my neck. "We make beautiful babies, no?"

I stop rinsing. My stomach flip-flops.

Back in 1970, it took getting fired from Sambo's for me to admit that I was indeed pregnant. Somehow I had managed to ignore all the classic signs: no periods, swelling breasts, morning nausea, writing all of it off to exam stress and poor diet. Finally I went to the university clinic and was referred to several doctors who, though chancy, might still be able to help.

Mike drove me from Portland over the border into Washington, to a quonset hut on the outskirts of a small town where Dr. Greenbaum and his one-man, two-nurse clinic did abortions, inexpensively, fifty weeks of the year. He told us that he felt duty-bound to be available to the women of the Northwest; his daughter had died of an illegal abortion in Kansas several years before. His two weeks of vacation — one in summer and one in winter — were spent sipping mai tais on a Waikiki beach. The rest of the year, he said, was business as usual. He also said I was pretty far along and there was some danger, and I should think the whole thing over. Mike and I took a cheap hotel room not far from the clinic in order to sleep on it. Of course, we hardly slept.

"In our own way," Mike promised me that night sometime around four a.m. "With our own vows. For as long as we love each other."

It's hard to believe now that marriage was as unpopular as it once was, but in 1970 no one we knew had even remotely considered the idea. Mike wanted both to have the baby and get married. I could graduate, deliver in late summer, and we could get a farmhouse near the beach and live on food stamps until we decided what to do. Besides, he urged, marriage and a new baby would be more fodder with which to fight the draft board.

We went back to the doctor the next day — for blood tests — and were married in the town hall by a justice of the peace.

Just before I said my "I do" I looked across at Mike — blond and blue-eyed — and I compared him to Ole. Despite their radically different haircuts, I noted, with some relief, their features and coloring were fairly similar. In some way, they could have been brothers.

Dinner with Maxine and Nadi is interesting: tofu, seaweed salad, and a wonderfully rich nut and date desert that Nadi has made himself. Henry, as usual, insists on doing the dishes, and with Nadi drying, Maxine and I have time to ourselves. Outside on the wee deck overlooking a deserted parking lot, I assure her things are better with Henry.

"He's a catch," she says as we re-enter the kitchen. Both hands submerged in dishwater, Henry wrestles a wok while he and Nadi discuss the U.S. immigration policies for Middle Easterners.

"I have this killer itch," Henry says to me, smiling. "Could you help me out, babe? Right there, in the middle of my back."

I scratch. Despite both the warm weather and heated kitchen, I feel the muffler beneath his shirt.

On the way back over the Bay Bridge, Henry starts the conversation I've been skirting for weeks. He's driving his pick-up; we've been unusually quiet.

"Is this still all about the rally?" he says. "Because if it is, football season is practically over. No more lonely Sundays, I promise."

I don't know how to tell him that my Sundays haven't been lonely, so I say nothing, stare out the window. Moored out in the bay huge tankers lit with flashing red and white lights are reduced to tiny toy boats.

"What's really the matter, Kate? What's going on with you?"

"Nothing," I say abstractly.

"Come on. You hardly talk to me at work. You're always busy after work, and I can't say you've been very happy to see me when we do get together." His head swivels back and forth, so out of the corner of one eye I can see his blue ones probing me for response. He sighs, brings his shoulders to his ears, rolls them back. It's a gesture of both surrender and annoyance. I turn and set my hand on his thigh, kiss his arm before resting my head against his corduroy covered shoulder.

"Do you think we should stop seeing each other for a while?" he says, hesitantly. "Is that it, babe? Do you want to take a break or something?"

I slip my hand under his arm and hold tight.

"No," I say. He lets out a breath, relief.

"Do you want to get married, babe? Maybe we should get married?"

That summer of 1970, after Maxine was born, Mike and I raised bees and goats, sold honey and milk to our friends and neighbors and tried to pretend we loved the back-to-nature lifestyle. Two years down the line we finally admitted our mistake, first to ourselves and then to each other. Mike wanted to move to Vermont, back to his family; I wanted law school at Berkeley. We amicably split the household goods, sold the bees and goats, and agreed upon a schedule and support for Maxine. There were no hard feelings but for some time — especially when I was struggling through law exams with a pre-schooler fighting for my attention every step of the way, I cursed both him and my own naïveté.

On Monday I come home from work to find Maxine and Miguel sitting on the front steps, animated and chatting.

"Hi," I say with false cheer.

"Hi," they say in unison, and then Maxine turns to Miguel and back to me. She knows something is up but she's not sure what.

"Mom — I mean, Kate — this is Miguel."

He smiles at me. He knows he's made points, that it wasn't his place to let onto anything before I came home. "I know," I say. "You coming up?"

"Not today," he says. This gets to Maxine; she figured I was talking to her.

"What's going on here?" she asks, her head wagging back and forth between us.

Miguel rises, stretches one arm around my waist, kisses me lightly on the cheek. "See you tomorrow." Those points he just made? He loses them in a big way.

In my apartment, Maxine is lying on the bed, watching me change from my work clothes.

"So you've been seeing him behind Henry's back," she says. "This is not at all like you. *God*, Mom."

"I'm not really seeing him," I say.

"Come on," she says. "I wasn't born yesterday."

"I know very well when you were born." It's my mother-voice.

"Oh, *Mom*."

I start into my jeans. Halfway in I back out, opt for the comfort of sweatpants.

"What's wrong with you?" I ask. Max is staring at me, shaking her head. It's a mother's gesture, a mother's *tsk-tsk*.

"I mean, it's kind of dishonest," she says. "Not just to Henry. I mean, it's like you have a secret life. It's like I don't really know you. How many other lovers do you have?"

I'm looking at her eyes: blue and clear and trusting. For my daughter things are somehow simple, like for Miguel. When the replica of the Vietnam war memorial came to town, Maxine and I went to see it together. While I searched the wall for names of my college friends and grade school sweethearts, she stood back fifty feet taking in the full effect.

"I wouldn't have gone," she said. "I would have refused to go. All of them. They could have gone to Canada, or Mexico. They'd still be alive."

Tears dripping down my cheeks, I pointed out names to her:

the kid who grew up on the next street over, the guy in my freshman ceramics class. My hand passed over Ole's name, once, then twice.

"I knew him, too," I said, fingering the letters of his long Norwegian surname. "In college, we dated." Maxine was incredulous. "You dated a Marine?" she asked. "A *Marine?*"

"I'm late," I tell her now.

"For what?" she clips.

"Late," I pause. Hold her eyes with mine.

"*Late*, late?"

I nod.

"Oh, Mom." The hardness has left her voice. "Whose is it?"

"It doesn't matter," I say. "I mean, I don't know for sure."

I look away from her, into the mirror, but there I see her looking at me, at my back, shaking her head ever so slightly.

"I'll go with you," she says. "I mean if —"

I shake my head. No. Then yes.

Maxine moves to my side and slides her arm around my back. I rest my head on her shoulder, the lump in my throat rises, the tears come. I'm planning to tell her. Everything. About Miguel and Henry, and maybe Ole, too. But I know, even as I make this plan, that I probably won't tell all. My decisions have been too complicated even for me to make sense of. And I, a lawyer, know there are loopholes everywhere, things you can never know, the facts aren't always clear, the choices are not always simple. Maxine has both her arms around me. My head is against her shoulder. For the first time, I realize she is taller than I am.

TORTOISE HUSBANDRY

S he has dumped you, not without warning, but it still feels unexpected. And you are feeling lightheaded, your stomach a pit of snakes, as if you had downed ten cups of coffee. But you haven't because you basically aren't eating or drinking anything: The Misery Diet. You imagine you could make a lot of money if you published it in supermarket size. Acquaintances say you are looking wonderfully slim, and your friends urge you to eat. One lures you with bait of fudge pie, but you think now is as good a time as any to lose those fat and happy pounds that crept on in the last two years of what you now think of as your fat and happy relationship. Besides, her new girlfriend is thinner than you are. This makes you cry, and you wonder: If crying burns up calories and a body is made of mostly water, how long will it take to cry off ten pounds?

But you know all this because — most likely — you've been dumped before. But I didn't know it because I'd always been the dumper, not the dumpee. Smart, I thought. Only I'm not sure. Because if I'd had some practice I wouldn't be so inexperienced now. Maybe I wouldn't be so crazy or be doing such crazy things. In fact, I'm doing anything not to feel like someone has driven me blindfolded down a long and windy one-way street full of pot holes and left me at the end, precariously balanced on a cliff. In front of me stretches the grayest, bleakest sky I can imagine and this is Life. Mine.

So I'm taking showers at five o'clock in the morning. Long ones. I wake up suddenly, knowing she has just turned toward her lover in bed — the same way she used to turn toward me around five. I sit in the shower, using up all the hot water, and I'm momentarily comforted. My utilities bills have almost doubled.

And this new pet idea. Not a cat or a dog, or anything warm and cuddly. No, a small reptile that my mother has procured for me. In her conservation group, my mother discovered the plight of the endangered desert tortoise. She herself has adopted a flock of these small reptiles as part of a bid to revitalize the species. She got an extra for me.

"A pet that will last," she said on the phone. I started to cry again.

"Drive down for a visit," she said. "I've got a tortoise right here with your name on it. A change of scenery will do you good."

I whimpered my agreement into the receiver.

My mother, a widow, has been very kind throughout this breakup, but really she doesn't quite understand. She and my father stuck through thirty-five years of marriage and since he died she's dated, but nothing serious, or as she says, dramatic. She saw me leave my last lover of two years for this one, and so she wasn't surprised to see this one leave for another. For some time I assumed this lack of total compassion was because of me being gay, but now I think it's because to her, thirty-five years of marriage seems like a relationship and anything else seems like dating. My girlfriend Stephanie and I didn't have kids or a house so our break was clean and fast, not as complicated as a divorce. We returned all borrowed books and clothes, but that was during the first days of shock when I was amicable and not the madwoman I've become.

It's a five hour drive south to L.A., through the vast dry countryside that is central California. The somewhat nauseating smell of livestock punctuated the miles of emptiness. Roadside service stations and garish fast food places splashed the only color onto an otherwise gray and brown landscape. During the drive, I daydreamed of Stephanie and eventually cried myself out. I arrived at my mother's red-eyed and ready to meet my pet.

A rocklike object, slightly pungent though not unpleasantly so. I took the small animal in my hands and kissed the hard shell of its back. It peed on me. "A reaction to danger," my mother said and I thought, *not a bad one.*

After a week, during which time I cried, rested, ate tiny portions of chicken soup, ran up my mother's phone bill with calls to my therapist, and watched daytime soaps (which made my life seem, if not simple, then downright predictable), I put the tiny tortoise into a cardboard box and announced it was time to head home. It was late March and the nursery where I worked said they wanted me back, since people were gearing up for spring planting. As I readied to pull out the drive, my mother handed me a file folder an inch thick labeled "Tortoise Husbandry."

"What are you calling it?" she asked. I picked up the turtle and he drew his limbs inside.

"Touchy," I said. "Because every time I touch him he disappears into his shell."

"You won't actually know if it's a 'he' or 'she' for about ten years," she said.

The idea of that many years of not knowing anything made me start crying again. I pictured us living together alone in my small apartment. My only bed partner a cold-blooded asexual reptile. I sniffed and set Touchy back into the box.

"Good-bye Touchy!" My mother waved me down the street. As I turned the corner she was still waving. I negotiated the freeways out of L.A. in a daze, which is probably the best way to do it.

I had planned to get home that afternoon. Get back to work in the morning. But as I drove out of the city I found myself wanting to take the long way. Why rush? At least in Atascadero I wouldn't run into Stephanie or her new girlfriend, Annie, or any of the five hundred other lesbians who were privy to my drama.

As I drove I imagined all kinds of things. Dying was on the top of the list: Wouldn't she be sorry then! Or perhaps I would get those leather pants; I'd be irresistible. She'd come crawling back. Everything I thought of was to keep out the memory of her on top of me, her long brown hair tickling my ears, her fingers inside me and her voice, "Uh, huh, come to me baby . . ." I felt sure I'd never have sex again in my life, or if so, it would never be as good. So what if we fought before and after?

Touchy rattled around in the box. I tried to take the curves slowly. The sky was low and gray, the road almost free of traffic. I struggled to keep my mind off Steph. I sang along to bad country-western. But each tune seemed to capsulize my life: "You're gonna crrryyy, over all the reasons whhhyyyy . . ." Or, "I'm addicted to you baby, you're a hard habit to breeeakkk . . ." I switched off the radio. Touchy moved around in his box. I guessed he was hungry, having no need for the misery diet. I decided Touchy was a he: I'd had enough of girls for a while.

In San Luis Obispo I pulled off and found a park. I set the

tortoise on the lawn where he chomped some grass and several clover flowers. Next to the park was a church and a spotted sign which read "Catholic Charities Thrift Boutique." When Touchy had finished eating (a moment hard to distinguish from resting between bites), I tucked him back into the car and wandered over to the church.

A small room was jammed with piles of clothes, dishes, books. A skinny woman in a pink sweat suit seemed to be trying to make sense of the jumble. "Can I help you find anything?" she said.

Looking around, I wondered how that could actually happen. "Just browsing."

"Feel free," she said, smiling.

I came across a box of glasses, forties cocktail tumblers, frosted, six in perfect condition. "How much?" I asked, opening the box flaps to show.

"Umm." She considered the box for two, three seconds. "How about a dollar?"

In my gentrified neighborhood these would have been at least twenty-five bucks, maybe more. I nearly forgot about Steph. In less than an hour I had amassed quite a pile: TV trays, old children's books, a wonderful fifties party dress (Steph's size), a vintage cowboy shirt, a martini shaker festooned with a topless go-go dancer whose hips moved with each flip of the glass. I was still full bore when I came across a nightgown, a Lanz nightie, like half the world wears, only it was the same pattern and style as the one Steph wore. The tears threatened. My stomach flipped.

"How much for this stuff?" I asked quickly, not wanting to make a scene.

"Five sixty-five," she said, after a moment of figuring. "Did you take a look out back?" She waved a bejeweled hand towards the back door. "That is, if we haven't yet cleaned you out."

I made my way to the back of the room and pushed the door. There were several piles of clothes on the ground, a jumble of rusty bikes against the side wall. And then this large sofa. Fifties, a kind of blue, with sloping arms and a quilted back. I'd been looking for a sofa. Indeed just three weeks ago Stephanie and I had shopped for a sofa. That was the day she told me about Annie.

Tears again. The pinched heart. I went back inside.

"How much for the sofa?" I asked just to break the sound of my sniffling.

"That blue one? Take it, it's yours. A bonus for being such a good customer." She was wrapping the last of my purchases in newspaper. Three full grocery bags were lined up near the front door.

"I'm in a VW," I stammered. "And I live in San Francisco." But by then I couldn't believe my luck. It would look perfect in my apartment: a sea-foam couch with my pale pink rug. A new look. Fifties. The cocktail shaker a perfect accent. Steph would be impressed. "But I suppose I could drive down next weekend, if you could keep it here."

"Well, there's not a lot of room here, honey. But I'll take it home, and it'll be there waiting."

"You would?" Small towns suddenly seemed like the place to live. Cheap thrift stores, free couches, friendly people.

"Sure, you look like you're having a rough day."

I nodded. "But things are looking up now," I said. We made arrangements and packed everything into the bug. Touchy had disappeared into a nest of newspaper.

I attempted to convince my best friend Andrea to make the trip back down with me. I promised an adventure, scenery, fresh country air. Nothing doing. I pleaded. I wasn't up to making the trip alone, the tears still came suddenly and without warning, and half my days at the nursery were spent hiding behind a rosebush, honking into a crumpled kleenex. She wouldn't budge.

But on Thursday night Andrea relented: Her sometimes wayward girlfriend had taken up with a visiting young and sexy British filmmaker — "Just for a week or so" — and Andrea was eager for any excuse to leave town. We made a pair: two morose lesbians toddling down I-5 in a borrowed pick-up. Andrea drove. I held Touchy. I was beginning to grow very fond of him. At night he made scratching noises, surprisingly comforting in the quiet of my apartment. In the mornings his ancient face watched as I chopped and sorted his day's rations of vegetables. He fit neatly in the palm of my hand.

I talked about Steph. Several times I had seen her car in my neighborhood. I thought she may have been checking up on me. I wondered if she wondered if I was seeing anyone. Maybe it was her who called and hung up on my answering machine. I heard that the new girlfriend had been seen with her ex-girlfriend. I wondered if we'd be back together before my birthday next month.

We arrived around noon and got directions to the woman's house. It was out of town, on a dirt road, a small but modern house with a rusting swing set in the dusty front yard. I left Touchy on the floor of the cab and Andrea and I carefully avoided the dog droppings which polka dotted the path to the front door. At the sound of the doorbell there was a huge uproar: yelps, barks, snarls. A minute later the door creaked open and a couple of puffy eyes peeked around the edge.

"Down Reggie! *Down!*"

Andrea stepped back right into a semi-atrophied pile of shit. "I'm here for the couch," I said as Andrea pawed the dirt.

The door closed and I heard the dog being dragged to another room. Then a huge hulk of a boy stood suddenly before us. He was over six feet tall and wore rumpled green pajamas with a sleeping bag draped over his shoulders like some sort of Superman cape.

"Mom's sleeping," he said. "But come on in and get it." He opened the door and we found ourselves in a dark living room shrouded in a TV glow. A man holding a beer sat in a lawn chair in front of the TV. It looked as if there was a fresh wound over his right temple. Several bodies were intertwined on a ratty sofa. Andrea leaned into my ear, "Let's go." I swatted her away.

"Dudes!" The big guy kicked the back of the sofa. "Get up! They're here to get the couch."

It took several seconds for me to realize what had been implied. That ratty sofa was *my* ratty sofa. In the half light I could barely make out the color: a washed-out blue, tinged with yellow. I stepped forward. The arms were fuzzy and frayed, clawed by cats.

The two bodies unwound, and a girl and boy ambled out of the room.

"Hey, Pops, give us a hand."

The man set down his beer and stared at the boy as if to place him, then rose and clapped his hands together. He wiped the back of his hand across his face and a streak of blood striped his wrist.

"Got hit with a pizza box," he said when he noticed me staring. "Almost took my eye out." The father and son each took an end of the couch and hoisted it up and out the front door. The dog started barking in the next room.

In the afternoon sun, the couch was a puke blue-green with

large patches of browny-yellow on the back. For a minute I thought they had ruined the sofa somehow in the last week, but as I got closer I could see that it had been deteriorating for ages. The stains were well seasoned, the moss-blue a very distant echo of former beauty.

"Won't stay like that," the man said balancing the sofa in the back of the truck. "Got any rope?"

"We're not going far," I said and both man and boy gave puzzled looks. They knew I was from San Francisco. I didn't want to go into it. "Thanks," I said. "And thank your wife." The man ambled back into the house. The boy had repositioned the sleeping bag around his shoulders and stood there in the mid-day sun like some sort of modern totem.

"It's awful," Andrea said as soon as we were both in the cab. "I can't believe you thought it was worth anything. It's ugly and stained and old and —"

"Okay, *okay.*" I sat in the cab holding Touchy. "What are we going to do with it now?" It was dreadful. More than dreadful. And I couldn't believe I had thought otherwise.

We stopped at a telephone booth in town and tried to locate a dump. No dump. Then we called the upholstery shop and asked if they wanted an old sofa. No, but they told us of a thrift shop in town that took just about anything. By the park, in the back of the church.

"Yes, I know the one . . ."

We unloaded the sofa, set it up against the building just by the back door. We grabbed some burgers and were back in the city before eight.

As we rounded the corner onto my street I saw Steph's car parked near the corner. "She's back!" I said and peered towards my apartment. "I think there's a light on —"

Andrea stopped the truck, reached across the cab and put her hand on my leg.

"Steph's moved in with Annie. Down the block. I didn't want to be the one to tell you but —"

My body went through its gyrations: heart pinched, pounding, a cold sweat. I let the tears come up and out.

"The sofa," I said, finally, and shrugged. "Hope springs eternal."

Andrea's touch warmed my leg. Touchy was cold between my hands. I kissed the back of his hard shell and closed my eyes. Worse things would happen in my life. Someday the sofa story would be funny.

I asked Andrea to stay the night. We watched late-night TV and cursed British filmmakers and everyone named Annie.

Evidence that things would get better.

II. Now This about That: Essays

WRITING OUT MY LIFE

I've been keeping diaries since I was nine when I first read Louise Fitzhugh's book, *Harriet the Spy*. This book changed my life. Harriet became my hero and my role model. She was a tomboy who wore denim trousers and carried a flashlight and a spiral bound notebook in which she wrote down everything about everybody. Harriet covered a daily spy route, jotting down important observations and detailing the often-puzzling behavior of those around her.

By the time I'd finished *Harriet the Spy*, I had purchased my first notebook. It was orange and brown paisley (*circa* 1967) and flipped open at the top. In Girl Scouts, I braided a lanyard and fashioned a short leash to secure the notebook to my belt loop. I carried this notebook everywhere. I slept with it under my pillow. On the first page I wrote "KEEP OUT! THAT MEANS YOU!" and drew a skull and crossbones. I recorded my first-ever journal entry: "Vincent has a hole in his pants right *there*."

I filled this notebook quickly with snotty observations: of my teachers ("Mr. Garris is a fox, Mrs. Zink obviously dyes her hair"); my friends ("Kerry is getting fat, Angel always smells like garlic"); and my family ("Gerald Rafkin is weird"). I dated the last page and quickly purchased another, with a cover of pink and Day-Glo green psychedelic waves. I drew pictures in this one, worms wearing funny hats, and scribbled poems. My favorite, "The Moon So Soon," a quatrain I wrote in 1969 about the lunar landing which ended, "When they're up there all night/I'm so very, very uptight."

I kept various notebooks over the next ten years. After a spate of small, spiral pocket-sized ones, I graduated to the new hardback "blank books." I kept a red one reserved for periods of anger, in which I used only red ink. My best friend and I had another in which we coded all the boys' names. Russel became "The Wind" because of "rustling through the trees." We named a hawk we spotted "Freedom in the Sky." Remember, this was 1974.

During high school I wrote in a formula book that my father had saved from pharmacy school. It was tabbed from A to Z, and there were recipes for various drugs scribbled on yellowed pages. I alphabetized my entries. In the "D" file was my diary; in the "B" file, boyfriends; in the "W" slot, all my observations on weirdos. "K" was for kissing and I wrote down the name of every boy I kissed and underlined those of note.

When I tell other writers that I have such a detailed record of my early life they are often jealous. I knew I was going to be a writer, and so I wrote. It was as simple as that. But most of the material in these early diaries isn't very useful. My observations were fairly mundane, my concerns — boys, dates, popularity, parents (yuk) — run of the mill. I have, however, been able to snatch the voice of my childhood and use it in my work, and even lift, verbatim, one short-short from a 1975 entry:

Why I'm So Screwed Up Right Now

Here's a summary of why I'm screwed up right now. First, I was supposed to like Chris, and I was informed by many he liked me. So, I went to the football game which we won. It was a really good game and I cheered a little. I thought that he would not be at the game because I was also informed that him and Steve were working. But when I arrived at the party at Jon Dik's they were there. Must have got off early. Anyhow, David gave me some beer. Like three bottles. I talked to Chris for a second, but I was too busy looking at Steve. Fuck! Did he look nice! Gina was talking to Chris and he (Steve!) walked up. So I said to Steve: You're the one who doesn't give anybody beer. And he said: Come outside and get some. So I did. Then we were going to come back in and I asked him if he was going to even be my friend. So he said yeah, and then he just put his arms around me. So I proceeded to say some things I shouldn't of such as: The only reason I liked Chris was because I was horny. And some other good ones like: I really like you and missed you so much when I was at camp. To that he replied: I heard about you at camp. But he wouldn't tell me what he heard. Then we walked back into the house. And I saw Chris and this is the only word that can describe what

I felt: Fucked. So Steve walked me home and I just let him sit on my front porch. I told him I was going to kiss him and he said: Who said you could? But I did anyways. Then he went back to the party and he told Gina that it was a big mistake that he walked me home. Also Chris couldn't understand why I was with Steve if I really liked him. I felt so fucked. Chris is such a neat guy. Tomorrow at school is going to be touchy. All I'm going to say to Steve is: I'm sorry for how I acted the other night, and if you want you can just forget it. To Chris I'm going to say: I'm sorry I was so screwed up at the party, I really didn't know what I was doing and what I was saying. I knew you knew I liked you and I do. (I'm only going to say this part if I know Steve doesn't like me.) Talking to Steve is going to be easy compared to talking to Chris. Anyway, that's why I'm so screwed up right now.

Scary, huh? I have a cardboard box jammed with twenty years of journals hidden in my basement. There is a note taped to the top of the box: "Read at Your Own Risk." Are they incriminating? Only to myself. Some future reader might have a heyday. More likely: drown in boredom. But still, these form a record of my life: who I was and what I cared about.

After I graduated from college with a U.D. (Useless Degree) I went to get an A.U.D. (Another Useless Degree), after which I found myself looking for work. I had called myself a writer for so long I thought it was time I did something about it. So I presented myself to several newspaper and magazine editors as one. To my surprise, they believed me.

Freelance writing has always felt to me like *carte blanche* to be rude. You can ask anybody anything, it seems, and if they are guaranteed a column inch they'll tell you. Ego. My publishing career started with this kind of work; everything I was curious about became a story. Did that slum lord really kick those senior citizens out onto the *street*? I am grateful for my curiosity, and for my naïveté.

My first book, *Different Daughters*, sprung from disbelief. I simply could not fathom what mothers thought was so horrible about having lesbian daughters. So I went and asked them. Sometimes I got answers I didn't want. I asked my own mother first. She asked back: "Why can't my kids be normal?" Other times I got asked questions I never expected: "Is there a difference between lesbians and feminists?"

Getting to ask anybody anything did not seem like work to me. Freelancing, I felt even more like Harriet the Spy than I did with that notebook swinging from my denim trousers. I was paid for being nosy, for asking hard questions. For seeking out my heros, having tea with them, and then opening up our conversations to the scrutiny of others.

I do less freelancing now, but my curiosity is still what sends me to the computer. I've written about everything from endangered reptiles to the fine points of afternoon tea to racism in the anti-racism movement. I've exposed local government overspending and crooked redevelopment schemes. Much of the time I've had a political axe to grind, if not wield. I write about what excites me, what confuses me, what I want to tell others, what I want them to believe.

But there are days when writing is hard for me. Weeks when I have nothing to say. I have a friend who claims that writing is her life, that it is what keeps her alive. If this ever was true for me, it isn't anymore.

To write you must believe you have something to say and ultimately believe there are people who want to listen to you. I'm a person who isn't set back too much by rejection. Those rejection notices that hiccough out of my mailbox rarely do more than scratch my spirit. By the time I've committed myself to paper, and worked something up until it's ready to go out, I believe it worthy of readership. That editors don't often just pisses me off.

But I've had lows in my life when depression, or drama and grief, or sadness keeps me from thinking past my own nose, let alone sending things into the void. Days when I don't feel good about myself, or the world, and can't imagine why I'd want to write anything to anybody, even a postcard. I've struggled with deep feelings of abandonment and loneliness and have awakened in utter despair. I'm not special. I'm no different from anyone else who hits these kinds of bottoms. I have childhood pain to deal with, and wounds of the heart. Some days the loss weighs me down like a cannonball in my gut. And when I'm low, real low, I can't write myself out of it, can't write myself a magic prescription.

Almost ten years ago I stood on a Berkeley street corner late one night arguing with my girlfriend. She was going through incredible pain, unearthing new memories of childhood neglect and abuse. She accused me of being unsupportive. "I've always been happy," I said, tasting the words like stale food as I spoke. "I don't understand what you're going through."

I'd just stopped drinking heavily and had not yet started to feel things deeply. I had yet to process my father's death and several other recent family traumas. But as I stood there watching this wonderful woman cry, a woman whose paintings captured a powerful depth of emotion that sprang from those very tears, I knew that I would have to start facing my own feelings if I was ever going to be any kind of writer. How could I write about pain if I couldn't allow myself to feel it?

But I was scared, too.

Several years later, during a particularly difficult time, a time in which getting out of bed, eating and sleeping were monumental tasks, when writing anything more than a check a complete impossibility, I came to the obvious conclusion that if I was unwilling to go through my own sadness, sadness would be something I could never write about. I had more information. I knew where sadness sat in my body, could feel the ache in my stomach, the tightness in my forearms. I could describe in my journal the four a.m. wake-up call that my heart sent out every night, a panic so deep that it opened my pores, caused sweat even in mid-winter.

I leapt into therapy, started to write in my journal, got a job writing radio commentary and eventually came back to function in the world.

My friend Michael, a poet, says: If you want to become a better writer, become a better person.

I have a quote of Nicole Brossard taped to my fridge. Brossard is one of Canada's foremost poets, a lesbian. She was asked what it took to write. Her response: "To respond to inner necessity — if only in self-defense . . . one has to want consciously or otherwise to make one's presence known. To declare one's existence . . . To write one must first belong to oneself."

During these times I pray for the return of that "inner necessity." Luckily for me there has always been a return, a replenishment. The depression melts, my curiosity and interest in the world slowly return, or my heart heals and an idea starts to stir in the same place where sadness reigned. One day I'll write an observation and stick it to my computer. The next day another will join it. Pretty soon there's a pile of notes, energy has amassed, and I'll want to move it. I'll want to write again. I'll want to surprise myself with what I know, and with what I don't yet know I know. This is the payoff.

And so I keep writing all sorts of things. Fiction. Nonfiction, reviews, and recently, a children's book. Sometimes writing makes me happy. Sometimes I'm incredibly uncertain about what I am doing. One of my friends, a successful novelist, says she is often approached by people who say they want to be writers. Her response: "So, do you like to sit alone indoors all day?"

Today is a gorgeous summer day in Provincetown. The beach will be swarmed with oil-slick tourists. It's so hot outside I'm naked at my computer. Later I'll swim. I happen to like my own company. If you want to write, that helps *a lot*. Most of the time, my projects amuse me.

Setsuko Migishi is one of Japan's most renowned painters. Now in her early eighties, her work was largely ignored in her lifetime. Recently there was a retrospective of her art at the National Museum of Women in the Arts in Washington D.C. The scope of the exhibit made me think about the reality of this artist's life. She literally worked for decades without notice. Because of this, her view of the artistic life struck me as particularly interesting:

. . . [T]here are peaks and valleys in an artist's life. Although there may be violent winds and snow, endurance and a life spent moving ahead and developing as a person are important. One must persevere. I believe that the most important thing, the greatest happiness for an artist concerns the question of how to lead a full spiritual life . . .

I have remnants of my early work, scrawled on the back of cocktail napkins: confessions of love and pain, superficial renditions of my chaotic life written in the daze of an alcoholic stupor. As a young dyke, I was a hard drinker. During this time I managed to produce a handful of stories, a sheaf of didactic political diatribes. I wrote a serial soap opera full of innuendo and gossip which was published in the local lesbian newsletter. None of this stuff was much good. I didn't know myself very well, didn't dive very deeply. I hope I won't live in that drunken place again. Knock on wood and offer a prayer.

And so I do the work, the introspection and, for lack of a better term, the self-improvement. I pay attention to my spiritual self. I meditate. I pray. These words look trite as soon as they appear on my computer screen. I read texts which help me connect with a larger sense of life. I study the *Tao te Ching*. I practice Poekoelan, an Indonesian martial art which has deep spiritual roots. Each time I train I am learning about myself.

Writing is like much other work: It is a way to leave a mark on the world. And ultimately this world is transient. Like Migishi, I have come to believe that my development as a person is what will ultimately sustain my writing. I know that my work will improve as a by-product of my spiritual growth. Sometimes a walk in the dunes pleases as much as a story acceptance. I am as apt to hang with pals as hole up and force an essay. And I wonder if I'll run out of things to say. A writing friend and I have mused over whether this is lack of genius: Will sanity and spiritual health relegate us to mediocrity?

I don't want to follow Virginia Woolf into the waves — unless it's only for a swim.

The work that I put out in the world goes mainly without me. I can be pleased or dismayed by the reception it gets. But my work is not *me*. Once my work goes out it has a life of its own. My life is still just *me*. Even after a wildly popular reading, I go home and I'm just me, alone.

And alone in my room, I am more content with who I am than I ever have been. I can see more clearly. I have to be able to see the truth, to be able to tell it.

I don't make things up. Those childhood journals contain no stories of dragons or fairy princesses, though there is one ditty about a talking squirrel. As a fiction writer I seem to be limited by my connection to what is. I'm amazed by people's lives and ultimately find them more interesting than any I've ever invented. About my short stories, I'm often asked, Did That Really Happen? At these times I feel cornered, transparent, not like a "real" writer. And I usually dodge the question. But yes. To me, or to someone, somewhere — even if only in my heart.

I've been writing as primary work for the last three years. There are times I scan the employment ads trying to figure out what I'm really going to be when I grow up.

Last year I went through a difficult time which lasted much of the dreary Cape Cod winter. I'm a California girl and this was my third (and last?) stint in this bleak, wet, deserted township. My heart was confused, my past came rearing up to shed its shadow on the present. My best friends had vacated to a warmer climate and many days I felt alone and sad. One day I received a postcard from my friend Will, who features as Lenny in one of my short stories, "Blueprints for Modern Living." He had moved to a new state, far away from where we both had lived and worked together for several years. He wrote to tell me that he had recently picked up the story again and that he still loved it:

> Do I like it because I can remember how flattered I was to see myself in a story? I like it because it's a good snapshot of how we were then. I like how my image comes out and I don't usually like myself in snapshots. And I like it because of how forever close it makes me feel to you. I remember one day we walked to Cody's for lunch and I had a secret, which I could barely get out, which was that my wife definitely had decided to divorce me. And I wanted to tell you and have you weep for me and embrace me and convince me I could still live. I wanted you to fix the hole in my heart and make my life new. But you didn't, you couldn't. You wrote that story, and in it you hugged me when I cried — what I couldn't manage in real life — and somehow the story became the cure.

What I write about in that story never did happen. Sure, parts of it happened to me, and to others, but I never went to a protest march with Will and never held him when he cried. I wanted to, I wished I could, so I wrote that I did.

When I read that story at bookstores I often cry. For those moments — the time when I wrote that I could hug Will, when I wrote truthfully about the pain in our lives, and for the moment in reading when I can deeply feel his loss and my loss — it's because of those moments I write. Sometimes I look up and some-one else is crying, too.

THE MINE FIELD
OF LESBIAN FASHION:
OUT? IN? OR INSIDE OUT?

W*rong,,*" Jackie said shaking her head. We had just worked out. I was putting on my sneakers, white Nikes over black and white wool argyle socks.

"No dress socks with tennis shoes," she said. "And your socks have to be lighter than your shoes. And with sports shoes the socks have to be cotton."

I sat frozen to the bench. Hadn't I read years of *Glamour* magazine's "Dos and Don'ts"? And hadn't I winced at the photos of girls in the wrong coats, carrying the wrong bags, layering the wrong sweaters, those photos of slight girls on windy New York streets with black brick-like bars slapped over their faces to save them from what could only be acute embarrassment? (What a way to show up in a national mag, I thought in my younger years when I sought fame: as a "Don't.")

But here I was, a lesbian voted "Best Dressed" of the 1976 Senior Class of San Clemente High School, IN THE WRONG SOCKS.

I had slipped. The black and white photo — a black slash across my face — the caption: "Dress socks with sports shoes? DON'T."

"But Jackie," I pleaded. "These are warm. And besides, they tie the white of the sneakers into the black of my jeans . . ."

"Forget it, girlfriend," Jackie said like the savvy New York dyke that she is. "Get yourself to the Gap."

The mine field of lesbian fashion.

It's treacherous. A constantly shifting battleground demanding changing strategies and perspectives.

Let's digress.

I came out in the early eighties, and I visited my first lesbian bar with much naïveté. Ronnie had just ridden his horse into the White House, and not coincidentally I was living in the Antipodes. Auckland, New Zealand. The circumstances around this first foray into lesbiana are a tad sordid. The scenario, briefly: a feminist arts festival, lots-o-lezzos trotting about, a girl who had gone out with a boy I was going out with. This girl in a lesbian rock group. Me: a groupie.

Question: Can I be in love with the ex-girlfriend of my boyfriend?

Answer: Sure, but she doesn't have to be in love with me.

She did, however, suffer me one deep kiss before suggesting that she show me the "Club." (I now understand why I didn't have a chance with her: Two femmes? A tricky situation for a beginner.)

I dressed with care, having no one to ask, no cross reference. How I wished I was back in high school with the old gang so I could call a pal: What are you wearing? I was in my late-punk stage, long curly hair, a stripe of red — geranium red — over one temple. After many changes of clothes, I set this coif against a torn t-shirt which featured black bombers silhouetted against a paint-spattered backdrop. My miniskirt: red-black and green. Finally, red pumps. Pointy, sixties retro. Inch-high heels. Lipstick to match. My roommates at the time — straight girls not unsympathetic to my experimentation — approved enthusiastically. "You look hot," Julie said. I should have been suspicious of such support.

I trailed my crush up two flights of an old warehouse. The downstairs was home to a body shop and the second floor reeked that particular oily New Zealand smell of shorn sheep. At the crest of the last flight of stairs sat a table surrounded by a flock of slick women smoking Marlboros and collecting "dues." The "Club" was known to all outsiders as The Inner City Women's Recreation Group, and membership was private and by invitation only.

After I paid my three dollars, I shuffled into a large, dark room with a disco ball spinning in the center. On one side, a low-hanging light flooded a pool table. In a corner, a table behind which liquor bottles and crates of beer were stacked. A gaggle of girls danced cooly to the Eurythmics. Another group surrounded the bar. At our entrance it seemed as if everything stopped. Everyone turned and stared. My date (a misnomer I soon found out) disappeared into the dark, and I was left standing against the wall feeling like I did in seventh grade at my first dance when I had finally convinced my mother to let me shave my legs and wear "hose," only to find the other girls in hip-hugger corduroy trousers.

So here I was again, the only one in a dress, not to mention make-up. The swarms of jean-clad, sweatshirted, army-booted dykes circled with some disdain (distrust of straight women in those days was fairly rampant) before a brave butch soul asked me to dance. Okay, sure, we got together, but not for a few weeks and not until I had cut my hair, purchased black jeans, high tops, and a motorcycle jacket.

They say timing is everything. Now that skirt ensemble would be just the thing for warm summer night cruising.

Six months after I came out, my mother came to visit. She stayed in my six-dyke, multiracial, intergenerational, vehemently political, anti-everything, collective, vegetarian household. She gave it a good New England go. She asked me why we all "looked the same, like boys."

"We do not look like boys!" I countered. We were sitting on the front porch giving each other haircuts. The buzzer was out, everything from the ears down was coming off everyone, topknots were left, and "tails" snaked down each back and were wrapped with colorful thread or beaded. I'm somewhat shocked to notice that now, over ten years later, this haircut is sported by nearly every junior high kid I know. Dykes on the cutting edge?

But, I digress. We did look a tad like boys. Cute boys. And for several years we stomped around and kicked up enough trouble to keep us all bouncing in and out of court. We certainly did not ever want anyone to think we were straight. No, we didn't want to mimic any standards of traditional feminine beauty. (So we mimicked Michael Jackson and David Bowie instead.)

A year or so later, gals started wearing a spot of eyeliner — an especially nice complement to leather and studs — and pretty much all you saw on anyone was black highlighted by glints of metal. Not long after, I moved myself stateside, to San Francisco, where the range of lesbo fashion sent me reeling. I marched into my first dyke bar in black regalia only to find myself amidst — what? straight girls? Nope, femmes! Beautiful Latina women in clothes from Macy's and long fingernails — at least on most fingers

. . . And a gang of softball dykes, who looked like they leapt out of an L.L. Bean catalogue. You even saw older gals in polyester pantsuits with butches in men's trousers. Young punks in long underwear leashed — often literally — to girlfriends in little more than rags and safety pins. Gadz: Anything was possible. What was a young dyke to do?

I'm not such a young dyke anymore, but still my fashion dilemmas haven't been solved. And in some ways they get more complicated. I think the hows and whats of dyke dressing are always mitigated by bigger issues: Where do you live? How out are you? Do you want people to know you're a dyke? Are you dressing as a dyke among dykes or a dyke among straights?

My little town is so queer that many of these questions become twisted. Provincetown is a place where anyone can be anything and there is certainly one of *everything*, from the boy-toy clones to the drag stars to the straight men who come for the cross-dressing weekend (usually dressed identically to their wives). Fashion is something that gives shape to the gay parade each warm summer night.

I can dress completely "straight" here — in fact I now look more "mainstream" than I ever have, because no one assumes heterosexuality. Many of us locals have long hair, wear dresses and make-up. And when the gal touristos descend in droves, we're always amazed at how "dykey" they look. Everywhere there are music festival t-shirts and Girbaud jeans and high-top sneakers. There are jock couples in matching neon shorts and school teachers from the Midwest in khaki safari pants. Is there anything wrong with a lesbo look? No. And I can guess that in their hometowns such dressing is a clue to others, an underground code. The short-back-and-sides haircut of the bus driver is a message to the short-back-and-sides secretary. But here in Queersville not much of this seems necessary.

The most popular t-shirt slogans this past summer were "Nobody Knows I'm a Lesbian," and "I'm Not Gay But My Girlfriend Is." These eerie statements were printed in six-inch letters on the front of said shirts, and worn, I can imagine, only while here in P-town. Back home in Anytown I'm sure the slogans are all too real since — usually — people *better* not know. Fashion has to do with political choices; what's out or in has to do with one's own out-ness or in-ness, and where the political climate is swaying.

In many ways it was much easier ten years ago when my choice was limited to black, and my wardrobe consisted of three pairs of jeans, in various stages of decay, complemented by a purple "DYKE" button. I never wore a bra and hardly thought that years later I'd be going out dancing in one! But with all the choices available to me today, I'm often in a quagmire. What's a girl to wear?

My final digression: I have this unbelievable Polaroid picture dated on its curling edge July 1969. I was ten years old in this picture, taken at a summer camp carnival. I'm holding a stack of straws which I remember to be pea-shooters. And I'm dressed in this very strange get-up.

I had decided I wanted to be "half girl" and "half boy" for the occasion. The outfit is exactly that. On the left side I'm a girl: I've got a skirt fastened on one leg and a pink polyester shell that shows just the bud of a breast. My long blonde hair is wavy and loose, and red lipstick is carefully portioned over half of each lip. On the other side I've done the boy thing: a black vest, tight jeans, a single cowboy boot, my hair slicked back tight against my head. Both sides of me, girl and boy, are grinning wide.

In some ways I've spanned both sides of that early view of what I now see as my nascent lesbianism. I do the boy thing, I do the girl thing, I even do the cowboy thing. But, according to Jackie, and I'm apt to trust her, I still wear the wrong socks.

AFTER THE FALL

Two weeks ago I sat at my kitchen table talking with one of my best friends, who also happens to be an ex-lover. This woman and I are to each other as much or more than family. Our lesbian community is made up of many such relationships. We can't afford to run off and hide after each failed affair. Nor do we want to; the pain of that loss is far too great. There are new partners for both of us now, two years after our breakup, but we are still a very big part of each other's lives.

We were drinking coffee and talking. A spring rain had refreshed the struggling flowers in my window boxes. Another winter — Northern California style — had passed. We talked about our mothers. I had just started to realize that the delicate balance between my mother and me would soon topple, change into something I had only just begun to imagine. She is aging.

I'm just over thirty and my mother is nearing seventy. Given her good health, it is hard to see those years. She's a Southern Californian widow: jogs three mornings a week, walks on the beach, eats health foods, and square dances with the zeal of a high school cheerleader. She is nothing like her mother was at seventy: matronly in black dresses, infirm.

This conversation took place in my kitchen around three-thirty in the afternoon. I was talking about writing about my relationship with my mother; we travel together, we camp together, we go fishing together (although this last summer I noticed she would no longer take the steep paths down near the creek for fear of slipping). We are learning from each other and still learning about each other. After some years she has come to accept my lesbianism — my lifestyle she calls it — and respect my decisions, participate in my life, have relationships with my lovers and friends. In some ways I am trying to be like her and in other ways I fear our similarities. As in any mother/daughter relationship, there are complications.

After the rain stopped, my friend got into her utility truck and drove back to her job fixing appliances for PG&E. I made some notes in my journal — "immortality," "feminism," "community." And I went off to the newspaper where I work the swing shift. That night I came home to hear my brother's deep voice wavering on my answering machine: "She'll be all right," he first assured and my limbs went cold. "This afternoon, around four, Mom fell and broke her hip." He left numbers to call.

I froze, unsure, as if my conversation had somehow caused the fall, yet knowing that was impossible. For the first time I thought of my mother's death. Would she make it through a major operation? Would she lose her mobility? Her independence? Then I dialed frantically: my brother, her friends, the hospital.

Life would go on, I was told, only more slowly for a while. Mom needed care.

My brother was due to get married in less than a week; his honeymoon would follow. After the hip operation, mother would need someone full-time in the house. To pick up and go home seemed the only choice. I couldn't imagine a nurse, a stranger in our home, although I also couldn't imagine me moving back to the small and conservative beach town of San Clemente. My life was flexible, I had some time off coming to me, and I was caught up on my bills. Even so it was difficult to arrange the finances and logistics. What do other people do? People who don't have back-up and flexible jobs? Women who have families to support? Children who have moved far away from their parents?

Our country has no plans for looking after the elderly. My mother is lucky. My life has afforded me the time and luxury to set my Bay Area schedule afloat: I told work, teachers, editors, friends, and my lover that I was going, and I didn't know for how long. It was romantic almost, that shirking of responsibilities, and no one dared press me for a return date. I wondered if it's a kind of guilt that kept them from asking: I was the dutiful daughter, a shining example of child/parent devotion.

And so it was as if I'd been picked up from that kitchen table conversation and dropped into my hypothetical ponderings. I am taking care of my mother. I am in my mother's house, the house I grew up in. The neighbors come by, the same ones that carted me to swimming lessons, watched me build sand castles. Their kids and grandchildren come round. All make their way down the hall into my mother's bedroom where she reads, works crossword puzzles, rests, holds court. It is late afternoon and I just checked in on her. She is sleeping, her browned skin slack, weathered and rich against the white and lace of the sheets.

By all accounts she is doing marvelously. Nine days ago she couldn't walk, and now she is creeping around on her walker and taking short rides in her wheelchair. But it is frightening to see her helplessness. My pillar of support.

My *mother*.

And having never been close physically, it is scary to be so intimate with her body. I need to help her to bed, to the bathroom. For her, too, this must be difficult. A strong-minded, self-sufficient woman with little patience for disease or illness, she has found herself at the receiving end of a situation she has always abhorred. There is a strange embarrassment on both sides. For the first few days she had jagged crying binges — partially due to the morphine. Anger and helplessness seeped out from behind her closed eyelids. I tried to comfort her, but her first reaction was to dry her eyes, point her chin proudly heavenwards, and announce, "I've just got to accept this. Whatever happens, happens."

I think there are fears, unspoken, on both sides. I am wondering about her old age. How will we deal with it? What will be my part in it? She too must harbor these questions. If she becomes infirm, where will she live? With whom? I can't imagine living at home with her, but a nursing home? The thought sickens me, and who knows the real cost? Social security hardly covers living expenses, and my mother's government health benefits, she is told, don't cover all her expenses — even though she is over sixty-five. (Thirteen weeks in a nursing home eats up the savings of half those who enter them. Medicaid only starts to pick up the bills when a person's total assets drop below two thousand dollars.) If I hadn't been able to come home, I am assured my mother would have managed with home help and the support of her friends. We're lucky. Privileged. This time, she has savings, I have savings, and her injury is neither drastic nor unfixable. In time, a hip will heal . . .

So many sneaking fears play in my stomach, my throat. I am scared of being orphaned on this planet, losing the tie that has always held me to a "home" regardless of circumstances. And I am also thinking for the first time about my own old age. Who will be with me? Who will rinse out my bedpan? A lover? An ex-lover? Children? Mine or whose? Will I even make it that far? Will the world?

There is so much death around us in the gay community, it's almost as if I've forgotten about old age. No one seems to get there anymore. Cancer and AIDS take those in their prime. In my mother's neighborhood these realities seem very far away. Her friends have aged, as they say, gracefully. The neighborhood grandmother is in her eighties. She walks daily to the corner mailbox, drives, and still bakes the best cakes in town. My mother's best friends, two women slightly younger than she is, race around with grandchildren and embark on world travels. They see each other every day for a walk, coffee, or dinner, and talk on the phone. One lives two doors down, the other less than a block away. And all three women have known each other for twenty-five years. I can't imagine finding two best friends so close by, but we moved here in the fifties, and mothers spent days together while kids and husbands went off exploring the world.

In my first blush of feminism I pitied these women — and my mother — the way they all were sucked into marriages and families without thought of their own fulfillment. But now I'm uncertain. I've grown to admire, almost envy them, the simplicity of their choices. At nearly thirty I am sometimes bound by my own disappointments and confusions; no babies, no picket fence, no husband. Choices seem overwhelming, to move here or there, have a baby, move in with my lover, start tracking a career, or live marginally yet creatively. My mother came into her current career through volunteer work and is now happy at her job, leading whale watching trips and creating marine ecology programs for children and the disabled.

One of her best friends recently retired, and after many years of separation her husband moved back into her home — as her roommate and best friend. The other friend volunteers as a teacher of English for recent immigrants. All three women have experienced the influence of feminism on their lives — and have come out satisfied with their lots. And as far as I can see, happy. I think about my peers, our introspective concern with divining our own destinies.

I'm thinking all this as I do the things my mother did for me: cooking three meals a day, washing clothes, cleaning the house, grocery shopping, errands. After less than a week the novelty of her injury has worn off, and at times I am almost resentful. I am also incredulous that these women — my mother — did this same work for twenty years without much acknowledgment or appreciation, let alone compensation. I remember her sitting down Sunday nights while the TV blared another episode of some Disney movie, her pencil scratching the weekly menus onto a small pad which she kept in the kitchen. Dinners, breakfasts, packed lunches, afternoon snacks. When I think of her sacrifice — which she claims felt like no sacrifice at all — I think about my own lack of patience, my selfishness.

I don't know yet how this will leave us, or change us, as mother and daughter. I know my mother is a fighter, but this is round one of a fight she will inevitably lose. Eventually my mother and I will talk about her death, or perhaps we won't. Sometimes I am afraid. And then I know we are fortunate: There seems to be money and time enough for us to work together graciously towards whatever the future holds. But nothing is certain. There are few models for this stage of parent/child relationships. I truly wish there were. At some point I will be set adrift, whatever that might mean. I will face more choices in my life than my mother ever did, and I hope I can turn out as happy, as productive, as unregretful.

I wonder what my life will look like at her age: a collection of friends, ex-lovers, memories. Happiness? Health? In the year 2031, what will define the scope of my life, my family, my freedom? And as I care for her, deeply, this woman who has been so important to the shape of my life, I wonder if perhaps I'll never know this special mother/daughter relationship from the other side.

The TV in her bedroom has just gone off; it is shortly before ten p.m. on a Sunday evening. She is nearly asleep and thrilled to be able to turn, if only partially, onto her side. Her hip is still quite sore, and neither one of us knows how long it will be until she can walk or take care of herself. I get her a fresh glass of water. In the bathroom, gleaming hunks of wire and plastic sit in a glass by the sink: bridgework, with teeth. I've never been privy to this sight, or maybe false teeth are something I have failed to notice about my mother. I try to take my eyes from the metal, turn on the tap, fill the glass in my hand. I remember her delivering to me countless glasses of water, setting them on my bedside table. I place the small glass on her table and then kiss her good-night. Then I turn out the light and walk up the same hall she did, so many times, so many years ago.

PROVINCETOWN DIARY
(At the Fine Arts Work Center)

You have a life. It may even be a big life.

Work: thirty, maybe forty hours every week. Friends: three to ten people whose voices you find on your answering machine weekly or, in times of crisis, daily. A garden: aphids to fight, snails to monitor. You have pets. You have a good dentist. A reliable haircutter. You have a lover. She also has a life.

You write before work, at night, on Saturday mornings. Sending out queries and stories with those fat return envelopes that bug your mailwoman because they won't fit back through the slot without crunching. When people ask you what you do, you name your paying job. Then sometimes, secondly — though you've been published, and though you've been paid, and though you've been doing it for as long as you can remember — you say, "Also, I write."

"Oh, really?"

You say, "Yes." Firmly. But inside it doesn't always feel like you're a writer. It's the paying work that takes the greediest bite of your time. That defines you in so many external ways.

But one day the phone rings and this angel on the other end asks you for a date: seven months on the far side of the country. On a spit of sand you've only read about in *People Magazine* following mention of the Kennedys. Cape Cod. It is morning in your Bay Area apartment; the neighbor's stereo is blaring, and a siren outside has encouraged the local pack of frustrated dogs to begin their daily concert.

"What?"

You won out over several hundred other applicants: You've got a slot at the Fine Arts Work Center in Provincetown. True. You fall to the floor with joy.

Then you call in sick. It's definitely time to use up that sick pay.

Massachusetts. (At first you can't even spell it.) The Fine Arts Work Center. A winter's worth of free rent, utilities, too. The only place in the country that provides long fellowships to "emerging writers." It's because you're a writer! Ha! You're a *real* writer. Your mother is astounded. She doesn't quite get it — you mean you don't have to *do anything but write?* She calls the relatives nevertheless.

Dump that daily grind of a job. Even a great haircutter can be replaced. (With some difficulty, it turns out.) A lingering good-bye to your lover. (That life she has? She doesn't want to leave it.) Seven free months at the tip of the world can't be passed up.

We arrive October first. It's clear and beautiful in Provincetown. By now the tourists have left and the leaves are beginning to turn. This California girl has never seen such a thing. Just like in the Kodak commercials. Sky divers of yellow and red.

We're shown to our apartments and handed checks ($375 for writers, a tad more for visual artists). As soon as I close the door I burst into sobs. It's not bad, but it's no palace. The second floor of a rickety barn that a realtor would graciously describe as rustic. Paint freckles the walls, green and black mostly, like some version of macabre measles. I can hear each footstep of my upstairs neighbor and the long, sorrowful sigh of the man below. No insulation. The places are supposed to be furnished, and mine is, in a fashion.

Several hours pass, by which time I've covered the ratty sofa with a favorite piece of fabric, tacked photos of friends and family above my desk, arranged for paint to cover the spattered walls. Dry eyes now. There's a no-pets policy, but I've managed to sneak in my pal Sparky, a California desert tortoise. A beloved state reptile back home, here he's an illegal alien. By the time I'm ready for the first of many unbelievable P-town sunsets, he's resting happily on his electric blanket, snoozing.

There are twenty fellows in residence at the Work Center, ten writers and ten "visuals" as they are soon referred to. Nearly all fellows live on "campus," in a scattering of buildings, studios, and a remodeled lumberyard near the center of this peculiar town.

Work Center life is vaguely similar to college. There's a communal mail room and nightly get togethers that may include popcorn and ping-pong. This batch of fellows is diverse, ranging in age from early twenties to mid-forties. It's mostly an East Coast lot with several Westerners thrown in. There's a bunch of M.F.A.s; only a few of us hail from the work-a-day world. Several are veterans of the fellowship circuit and know each other from here and there. There are couples and singles and single halves of couples. There are straights and gays and not-so-straights. New couples form and re-form during the long winter months. Thankfully, for the most part, we all get along.

At first the amount of free time is shocking. No work. No commitments to whomever or whatever. But we all slide into some sort of pattern. It seems the "visuals" tend towards late nights, even all-nighters, and the writers are more active during the day. Different parts of the brain perhaps? My downstairs neighbor is a seven a.m. starter. On a manual typewriter. I purchase ear plugs.

I tune into my internal clock. I wake late, nine-ish, breakfast with my boy Spark, and then work until two-ish on fiction. Afternoons I mail submissions and write nonfiction. Some days I don't write at all. I bike, visit new friends. Call on Ruthie at the local thrift store. Read. One week in February turns into a reading marathon. Sometimes I feel guilty about not getting enough done.

Around noon most of us appear in the common room mooning for the mail. Rejections are made more palatable when received in a crowd. They're compared and critiqued. In January, when the stunning autumn is just a picture postcard memory, and the snow and sleet keep us inside longer than we'd care to be, the mail lurkers are downright dangerous. But even those letters full of garbled news about life at my old work place begin to feel like reports from a foreign country. Most everyone in Provincetown is an artist or writer or both. No one you meet here ever asks if you have another job or what you *really* do. But January is hard. It is dark at four o'clock, and one day I'm shocked to find only a single shriveled zucchini at the grocery store. I'm told by the stocker, a poet, "Honey, if you wanted fresh vegetables you should have stayed in California."

Throughout the year we are visited by writers, big names and lesser knowns, some ex-fellows. Sometimes they look at our work or make suggestions. Sometimes they come to give a reading, schmooze, get away from city life. We eat potluck dinners and chat. Sometimes this is great. Sometimes it feels like no one really knows what we are supposed to do with óne another. The bigwigs aren't here as teachers, but certainly are not peers. Some contacts are made.

Still, much time is spent alone, though there is some exchange between fellows. We swap books, share rides to the nearby library, eat breakfast at the only restaurant that remains open year round. Friendships form across lines of art and literature. For the first time I feel like I'm beginning to understand something about post-modern art. We support each other as we start the spring rotation of readings and gallery shows. I join a biweekly writing group of locals, perfectly suited to my work and needs.

And I fall in love with the town. The way the postmistress knows me and will sometimes plant kisses on those hopeful submissions. The way straight and gay live alongside in nearly equal parts. Some of the straight fellows/fellas find the community a bit daunting (straight single girls discover the pickings slim). Of all the small towns in which to land, I've managed to set down in queer heaven.

People begin to grow anxious after the February thaw. What next? May looms. Fine to be a paid writer, but what gives when the gig is up? Like maniacs, we all submit for residencies, NEAs, teaching positions, whatever. Most apply for a chance at the second year fellowships: Two writers and two artists from all the fellows from all previous years get doled out another slice of pie. The applications are sent off-Cape to an unnamed jury. Some fellows get jobs at the local A&P. The stipends don't seem to quite cover the basics, let alone extras such as car expenses, phone bills, or even health insurance. Most fellows come with some sort of savings.

I've all but decided to return to my old job when the news comes in. I've been gifted another year! There are enviously spoken congratulations. Disappointments. I make plans for a work-a-day summer. On the last Saturday of April the visuals and the writers face off for a highly competitive game of softball. The visuals — who are that day being juried for their second year fellowships — run high on adrenalin and emerge victorious.

The next year passes alongside a new group of fellows. There's a different flavor to this group; they're younger and a bit more ambitious. I'm more integrated with the townsfolk now and some-times feel like a local. The year passes, much more quickly this time. Some days I have this sense that I have to write everything *now.* That I'll never get this kind of time again. And then other days I just walk in the dunes.

But now it's May and I've finally been given the boot. What really happened? I've completed a collection of stories, published a book of nonfiction and started a novel. More importantly, after fourteen months of being a named writer-in-residence I can see myself as one. Evidence: I declared "writer" on my tax return this year.

It's a shock to be paying rent again. No, I haven't left town. Provincetown is a hard place to leave. When spring comes around there are tulips everywhere. The box turtles come out of hibernation to sun themselves near the ponds at the National Seashore. It's a small seaside town without too many rednecks. Where else can you get all this? Sea, sun, even a super A&P. (Known — of course — as the Gay&P.) There's a flock of us ex-fellows in town. We work in restaurants and on whale boats and clean houses and complain about the tourists who pour down Commercial Street like lemmings. It's a life. A writer's life.

CLAMS FOR NIXON

When I was ten my world was full of sand and salt and endless days under the hot Southern California sun. All summer long I swam and rode the shorebreak on planks of hard-packed Styrofoam. My body was nut brown, and my face was streaked white with zinc oxide. Still, my nose peeled pink and by September was as rough as raw hamburger.

It was 1969, and elsewhere things were also hot.

In the heat, San Clemente's seventeen thousand residents were sleepy. Nestled halfway between Los Angeles and San Diego, this bedroom community was peopled by mostly white working professionals, couples who had come from far and wide to live by the idyllic Pacific. Hardly anyone lived more than a mile from the beach. There was a small Hispanic community in the south end of town, but the only blacks were those shipped in to the neighboring Marine base.

Though the town bordered Camp Pendleton, and young, shorn boys with southern drawls walked the beaches in their heavy fatigues, Vietnam seemed a long way away. My small beach town with its vaguely Spanish flavor had yet to appear on maps of California, and I think many believed that until it did we all were safe. The outside world was full of scary stuff, but it seemed our only taste of that world was provided by the few long-haired hippies who drove through town in battered VWs on their way to Mexico.

Life in San Clemente was sun and surf and cocktails at five. Small children built sand castles along the shore line and collected clams and small sand crabs with trowels and plastic buckets.

This is where the story starts, the story of me and Richard Nixon and John Ehrlichman. And perhaps it's connected to the story of how I ended up a feminist, driving a Honda slashed with faded Jesse Jackson stickers. You start out somewhere, by chance, and then you end up somewhere else.

127

Here is the story as best as I can tell it. I was ten, and I liked to go clamming. For those of you who haven't clammed, here's the run-down. Clamming's one of those terribly unfair hunting and gathering activities. My father would watch the tides, on the lookout for an extra low one. Then, on a Sunday, two or three of the neighborhood families would gather buckets and trowels and hand rakes, don pedal pushers, old sneakers, and straw hats and make our way to the clam beds. The beds were rocky tide pools at the south end of town on a beach in front of a private community. A friend would let us in through the guarded gate. We'd park the cars on the bluff by her house and climb down to the beach.

The trick was to uncover a nest of clams, or a vein, as my father would say as if we were prospecting. I used to hop from rock to rock, slipping in occasionally up to my knees, probing urchins and anemones and small frightened octopuses. I would try to think like a clam. If I were a clam would I like to live here? Under this rock? Or this rock? And I used to do all right with this method, finding my own veins, feeling somewhat guilty as I pulled and grabbed at the spitting clams. Whole families of clams filled my bucket. The baby clams, those under two inches and therefore illegal, were left behind to fend for themselves.

So we'd dig for hours, eat picnics of Wonderbread sandwiches and deviled eggs and drag the buckets — brimming with clams in salt water — back up the bluffs to the cars. Occasionally a ranger would drive up in a jeep and make us count them out — fifty per adult and child — to make sure we weren't picking the beds clean.

But then Nixon came to town.

Nixon moved in with great fanfare as realtors and businessmen looked on greedily. The mostly right-leaning town held gala celebrations. My fifth grade class made welcoming signs, and we were bussed the half mile to his helicopter landing pad to greet him on his first arrival. Somewhere there is great television footage of me in a chorus line of children holding signs which spelled out "Welcome President Nixon." I held the "X."

With Nixon in town, we no longer had access to the beach. Lucy Cotton — the friend who had always let us walk through her property — had sold her father's Spanish villa, to be converted into the Western White House (despite her father's Democratic leanings and great friendship with President Roosevelt). Nixon moved in a slew of Secret Service men who dressed in suits and brandished fishing poles, and who patrolled the beach with what I saw as an evil vengeance, confiscating the surfboards of those young men daring enough to paddle in from the public beach to catch the best waves in the area. As San Clemente hit the news and made the map, I, turning eleven, just could not believe we couldn't go clamming anymore. I couldn't accept it.

I sat down and wrote a letter: "Dear President Nixon . . ."

I told him about how we were friends with the people who used to live in his house, and I told him about clamming and about how there really weren't any other clam beds in the area. I told him how I had greeted his helicopter, and then I asked him if he would let us — my mom and dad and I and maybe some of the neighbors — cut through his property to the clam beds and if that was okay, could he tell his Secret Service men to let us onto the beach? I also told him I would teach him how to clam, show him where the best veins were, and then I included my mother's recipe for fresh clam chowder. I drew a bunch of clams dancing around the paper — they had long necks and wore high heels and bikinis — and then drew some more on the envelope and mailed it to the Western White House.

It only took a week to get a reply. A long white envelope arrived with a blue embossed return address which read: THE WHITE HOUSE. I opened it, a two-page typewritten reply! I was sure we were all going clamming. I quickly flipped to the end, to see the signature, and was startled. *Who was John D. Ehrlichman?* I didn't even get an answer from the President himself!

I think my father then read the letter, which though hopeful, disappointed me. I don't know why, I suppose because I had imagined telling my friends that I was a personal friend of the President or perhaps I thought I'd make the news strolling along the beach with Dick, Pat and full clam buckets.

The letter from Mr. Ehrlichman was itself quite something, but I didn't know that at the time. It was long and chatty and somewhat pathetic though I can't exactly say why. I guess because it was 1969 and a whole lot was going on. I imagine him sitting down in some office in the White House replying to a young girl's wish to go clamming, while in other offices plans for secret bombings were being drafted and carried out. In retrospect, it's a scary juxtaposition.

I believe Ehrlichman typed the letter himself; there are a few "whited out" mistakes, and no secretary's initials. It began by saying that the President asked him to answer me directly and then told me it was his job, as Counsel to the President, to ready the new property security-wise. It described the work being done — the construction of the swimming pool and windbreak — and then suggested that it might be possible for us to go clamming later in the summer:

> I think after we get out there this summer it might be possible for us to work out some way for you to get to and from the beach with your clam buckets (if you can work out something with the Secret Service so they will let you on the beach!) but I think that we had better wait and see how that all develops.

I wonder how he expected an eleven-year-old to work something out with the Secret Service? He went on to say that he would be very happy to see me if I would come and visit him. "Maybe at the same time," he wrote, "you could show me where I could dig some clams. I'm originally from the Pacific Northwest and am very fond of nice clams."

He then signed off, adding that the President thanked me for coming to visit him on his arrival.

Although I was disappointed, I wrote him back. This turned into my first experience with bureaucratic run-around. I have several letters from him that basically said he was too busy to clam but would still like to go at a future date. The last letter is dated October 10, 1969. The still heat of the summer had finally melted into a warm breeze of a Southern Californian autumn and I was back in school. Five days later I wore a black arm band to my sixth grade. It was the Vietnam War Moratorium Day. I was the only one in my grade to protest.

Something happened over that summer. I didn't go clamming with the President but I came to understand war. Several neighborhood boys were nearing draft age, and I remember learning that it was "lucky" my older brother had punctured eardrums and flat feet. Life outside our summer city was coming through harsh and violent on the nightly news: Martin Luther King was dead, so was Bobby Kennedy. There was that nightly body count at the end of each broadcast. I sat in front of the television eating meat loaf and waiting for "Gilligan's Island" or "Lost in Space." When the October moratorium was announced, I knew I wanted to protest.

My parents must have said it was okay with them because somehow I got a piece of black cloth and knotted it around my arm, above the elbow. When I walked to pick up my friend next door for school — a friend whose father was in Vietnam flying bombers — I was very nervous. I was singled out in Social Studies for an explanation, and I remember telling my teacher, Mr. Garris (who himself must have been not long past draft age) that I wore the band because I wanted the war to stop. He nodded and repeated, "The war to stop." My older brother skipped school altogether, ostensibly in protest, but I vaguely remember him going to the beach that day.

The editorial in the local paper lamented the "Campus Radicals" who were "blind to the world past the borders of the U.S." The editor described the fingernail torture in Vietcong prisoner-of-war camps. "While they talk of brotherhood and compassion [the communists] seek to wipe out the structure of laws, government and business that has brought a greater measure of justice and compassion to the lives of men than any other system ever devised." Certainly there was never a ground swell of anti-war protest in our town. One protest that summer attracted some four thousand mostly out-of-towners, "clad in everything from army fatigues and work clothes to see-through blouses and bikinis." They were met at the gates to Nixon's estate by two battalions of trained Marines and over a hundred sheriffs.

Other small protests were held in San Clemente that year, despite moves from the City Council to thwart freedom of speech and the right to assemble. I don't remember much about them. I started to grow up then, I think. My mother and father took a meditation course and worked on the teen drug hotline, while my teenaged brother took drugs. I fantasized about being a fashion designer and sketched girls in low-riding bell bottoms with piles of stringy hair. Watergate came down and few locals could believe it. Slowly, I found out who Ehrlichman was.

I never went clamming again, even after he left. They built a nuclear power plant a mile from the clam beds and that changed the temperature of the water. Nixon finally got himself a place in Manhattan. In San Clemente there are still streets named after him. Del Presidente winds through the south end of town, and few remember when it was Calle Fuente. Some locals are still fighting for a Nixon library or at least a monument. I can only hope neither eventuates.

Many of my friends still live in San Clemente, as does my family. I visit several times a year and usually fit in a walk down the beach to what the locals still refer to as Nixon's estate, although the grounds have been subdivided and developed into a sea of luxurious condominiums.

People often make fun of us So-Cal natives; we're thought of as conservative and right-leaning. People who meet me are surprised I grew up in San Clemente. But when I think of that summer of 1969 and the hope, naïveté and simplicity of my writing the President an invitation to go clamming, I don't think I've come so far. In '69 I believed wearing an arm band would stop the war. Ten years later I truly thought the ERA would pass. I couldn't believe it when Bush came out of the Iran-Contra fiasco smelling so sweetly — and still president. The world abounds with events that refute reason and fairness and grace. Twenty years later, I am still that little girl who refuses to believe she can't go clamming.

HOMECOMING QUEER

The announcement of a ten-year high school reunion made this ex-cheerleader shake to the soles of her Converse high tops. Time flies? Ha. My panic-stricken reaction: Has it *only* been ten years?

Imagine if you will a small Californian beach town. San Clemente's claim to fame is that it played host to Nixon's Western White House. To the delight of many and the chagrin of few, Nixon put my home town on the map — literally. San Clemente was and still is a Republican's heaven.

I went from kindergarten to high school with most of the same kids. Our parents met at the Alpha Beta and P.T.A. meetings, on the golf course or tennis courts, or at church. Presbyterians and Catholics. The first black kids came into town sometime during my high school years, and you could count them on one hand, not including your thumb. Gays? I thought they lived in nearby Laguna and were interior designers. I first heard of lesbians in fifth grade when Cindy Thompson ran up to me at recess, stroked my arm, and said "Lez-be friends." All the kids laughed. I didn't get it but laughed anyway. I went home and asked my baby sitter what it meant.

My high school scenario mid-1970s: The most important thing was to be part of the "V-squad." The V-squad was a band of ever-changing most popular girls who were "V" as in virgin. *Like* a virgin didn't count. Mostly we tried to go as far as we could without losing V-squad membership (round the bases but not hit home) or our boyfriends, football players and jocks. There were several social groups at school: sochies (socialites), jocks, nerds, druggies, and surf rats. Okay, I was a sochie, my boyfriend a jock — Most Valuable Player on the football team. I myself also qualified as a jock, being the only girl on the boys' water polo team. That presented a whole set of problems in itself: Pre-game pep talks in the locker room changed venue and, reluctantly, the coach made his talks a bit less spicy.

Getting dressed for high school was a two-hour ordeal: straightening and then curling the hair, changing outfits three times, calling to see what the other V-squaders were wearing. On game days we wore our cheerleading outfits and sipped soda cans filled with rum and Coke to give us that old school pep. Gossip and clothes were the (polyester) fabric of conversation, and gossip could be wrought from anything. After a Friday night, you had to re-convince the rest of the squad of your eligibility, even though the grapevine told otherwise. Beach parties abounded. Beach Boys, Neil Young, Cat Stevens, our soundtrack; Mustangs and Cameros, our chariots; Mad Dog 20/20, our drink. Sloe gin for special occasions. I can't tell you how strict the social code was: Popularity was measured down to the color of one's lip gloss.

So you can see I was thrilled for the chance to get together with the old gang.

I offer public appreciation to my friends who weathered my (several) apparel crises before the ordeal. It took hours of consultation to come up with linen trousers and a sequin-shell ensemble to highlight my flattop. My attempt to blend in was laughable as I arrived to find throngs of Dynesty-clad look-alikes in flower print dresses and frosted, lacquered hair. I was not only the sole female in pants, I was the only one with short hair. *Any* kind of short hair. No joke.

True to surf tradition, the boys' idea of dressing meant a new pair of cords and a Hawaiian shirt. The occasional "Miami Vice" clone stood out as spectacular. Girls who married outside the home turf dragged along well-suited, noticeably bored and uncomfortable mates who were then put on display à la gifts on "Wheel of Fortune."

Now several hometown friends had known of my coming out. My mother, who would have to face the aisle-to-aisle supermarket probings of small-town noseys, had balked at living with scads of inevitable town gossip. For the reunion we compromised: I wasn't allowed to don a label reading "Lesbian" (a fashion complement I hadn't really thought of wearing); however, if the subject came up, I could answer truthfully.

Before-dinner chat ranged from the kids to husbands, and only once did I have the chance to offer my status. Mostly I think people glanced at my left hand, assumed not married, and rabbitted on to tell the names and ages of their offspring. Many people had to get close enough to see my name card and its attached senior picture to recognize me. "I can't believe it's you!" they said fondly, remembering the Farrah Fawcett hair-do.

"I've been dreaming about this for ten years!" said the first drunken fool to grace the microphone. Our senior class president, aptly voted least likely to succeed, announced that he'd been trying to live up to that distinction since high school. I learned later that he has, having done time inside and a half dozen other things.

I sat with some members of the V-squad, long defunct, and their hubbies. I mentioned the girlfriend, received polite and seemingly-accepting approval. As more alcohol was ingested, responses changed. "Rafkin, you always did make us open our narrow minds. I'm just not surprised." Then an ex-cheer buddy asked me to dance. She kicked off her four-inch heels and bopped to a roaring Pointer Sisters tune. I'll be damned if she didn't flirt with me. My dancing was less relaxed than usual; still, raised eyebrows skirted the dance floor.

A "Magnum, P.I." look-alike surprised me with a hug and a kiss before I could recognize him as my very first ever boyfriend — fourteen years old and holding hands in a matinee, one kiss a day on the beach at sunset. Ah, romance . . . Having told me he'd spent half of his high school years thinking of my breasts and how elusive I'd been with them, he seemed most unnerved by news of my girlfriend. Somehow his dream had been shattered. I asked him for a dance for old time's sake, that is if he wouldn't mind dancing with a queer. "As long as you're not one of those male kind who always try to grab my ass." I assured him I wasn't and wouldn't.

Stray vixens roamed making stinging comments as they passed each other. "She certainly hasn't changed, still looks as sleazy as ever." Cliques re-formed with frightening ease. I chatted with the boys, feeling more comfortable talking of sports and jobs than labor pains and money market accounts for the kids.

Early on I spotted the other queer and later cornered him behind a fern. "Are you the other one in ten?" I asked nonchalantly, without a clue as to who he was. He looked startled, and I thought I might perhaps be in error. "You know, the other *one in ten*?"

135

"Um, yeah, I think, if I know what you mean," he stammered. "But *you?*"

We chatted, he wondering how I could tell he was one. (And we're talking obvious queer!) He conducts his life from a very small closet. Living at home, but not out to friends or family, on occasion he sneaks off to Laguna to hang out at a gay bar. Never been to San Francisco and couldn't imagine it. "A whole street of gay people, *wow* . . ."

I left as people started to stumble and plan the fifteen-year reunion. Singles and divorcees cruised the dance floor, chancing a shot with an old fling. I thought about what's happening in the world, the Supreme Court ruling against sodomy, about AIDS, about gay-bashing. I wondered about all the people who hate us: Were these them?

I thought about each one of us going to our high school reunions and coming out. Would this change people's attitudes? Would this challenge their hatred? In some ways I already live with their judgment, and this judgment is my own baggage. After all, everyone had been polite enough. Mr. First Boyfriend had even asked me sailing on his catamaran — no strings attached, he assured, glancing breastwards.

Or, had nothing changed in ten years? At the door I glanced over my shoulder waiting for the knives to hit.

SOMEONE EVEN MOTHER COULD LOVE

I want everybody's mother to like me.
That desire for acceptance is the complete antithesis
to the desire for change.
— Jewelle Gomez

About ten years ago I sat at my kitchen table with a shaggy collection of friends, lovers and lovers' ex-lovers, drinking beer and complaining about our mothers. What couldn't they *get* about us being lesbians? What was their *prob*-lem? We were baby dykes, young and confident and strong and in love with discovering ourselves and each other. Why couldn't our stupid moms see how great lesbianism was? For goddess' sake, why didn't they come out *themselves*?

Ah, youth.

No one was close with our families. We had little or no contact with our folks, or cordial but distant relations. Of the lot of us, I had perhaps the best relationship with my mother, but she lived seven thousand miles away, over two oceans, and had not laid eyes on me since my coming out. (Maybe she was a little afraid?!)

"My mom has never asked me *anything* about my life," Nina moaned. "Not even whether I'm seeing anyone." Nina had the dyke-cut of the day: shaved to the ears, a foot-long tail trailing behind, the top gelled to a scrambled froth. All of it dyed bright red.

"Well, mine was anything but supportive when Phillipa and I broke up," Krissy said. "She said something about it being 'too bad' and then went right on talking about how awful my brother's wife is because she's divorcing him. She's been cooking my brother breakfast, lunch, and dinner ever since his wife left him." Krissy smoked roll-your-own cigarettes and drove a hefty motorcycle.

Heather's mom lived nearby and visited our communal, collective, multiracial, vegetarian boarding house every few weeks. As soon as Heather spotted her mother's brown Rambler rolling down the lane, we girls raced around "de-dyke-ing" the house, stripping the walls of posters and photos, ensuring that everyone was dressed — preferably not in "Dykes Rule" t-shirts — and warning overnight guests that smooching was not *even* a possibility.

We tried to present a *nice* version of lesbianism, a version even a mother could love. I have to laugh when I look back at these attempts to make our lifestyle — wild haircuts and roaring motorcycles, and attitudes towards men that caused our mailman to shirk each day on his way up the path — palatable.

Collectively — and all projects were undertaken collectively in those heady days — we imagined a book telling mothers to accept their lesbian daughters. Here's what would we tell them:

Lesbians Are Great

We Are Nice People

We Are Not Child Molesters

We Want to Change the World (e.g. Overthrow Patriarchy)

Our Haircuts Are Not Masculine But a Response to Patriarchal Standards of Male-Defined Beauty

Not All Lesbians Hate Men

This last one we added as a P.R. move. The truth was, most of us had some "issues" with men. Those who didn't were too scared to admit it.

Our book would alleviate all maternal fear by answering all the Big Questions. Like, How Did We Become Lesbians? Few of us knew what to say to that. "It doesn't matter," Krissy decided. "Just write, 'We Are What We Are.'"

Rousing applause.

We even proposed to answer the oft-heard question, What Do They Do in Bed? However, we never really did answer that question since few of us had actually ever talked to each other about sex.

This How-To (Self-Help? Hardly!) book never did see daylight — thank god. We scrawled notes on the back of protest leaflets and stayed up late one night debating the cover design. Eventually I moved away from that gaggle of gals, grew up a bit, became slightly less self-centered. I began asking my mother what she needed to know about lesbians and learned that she needed me to hear her own feelings and fears. She needed validation as much as I did. So eventually I began to talk to other mothers of lesbians and to learn about their journeys towards acceptance and understanding. Because, like any dutiful daughter, I still wanted a book to give my mother.

I sent out flyers and posted notices asking for mothers who would be willing to tell their stories of how they came to understand their daughters. The first deadline passed and only a lone manuscript had found its way to my Oakland, California mailbox. After nearly two years of tracking, cajoling, pleading, scratching at leads and generally badgering a group of mothers to open up to me — a stranger — I finally had enough interviews for a manuscript.

Those interviews came together as *Different Daughters: A Book by Mothers of Lesbians* and six years later there are over twenty thousand copies out circulating in the world. Well, actually not all of those are circulating: I've received letters from lesbians who sent *Different Daughters* to their mothers, *certain* they tossed the book right into the trash.

But I've also received scores of thank-you notes, from mothers and daughters and even fathers who have found the stories in the collection helpful and validating. Today I came home to find a grateful mother on my answering machine: "I'd love to meet you; this book has helped me so much." How she found me I don't know. Letters come through my publisher, through friendly booksellers at stores where I've given readings. They're often on flowered notecards and range from simple thank-yous to heart-wrenching missives. "Will my husband ever talk to our daughter again?" one woman from the Midwest asks. "I'd love to correspond with you but only through general delivery — my husband must never find out."

These letters have continued to trickle in over the years, evidence that the book continues to lead a productive life of its own. Meanwhile, in the middle of my own life, my understanding of the book has changed.

Immediately after *Different Daughters* came out (!) I was barraged with requests for talk-show appearances, both TV and radio. Most wanted a mother/daughter combo. They sought palpable evidence of struggle and change; they wanted grimy details and *dish*.

"How could you, Mrs. Rafkin, accept your darling daughter — once a *cheerleader* — now a *lesbian?*"

"What went *wrong?* What do you feel when you see your daughter *kiss* another woman?" (What, was he *crazy?* I'd never kiss in front of my mother . . .) You know the questions. The kind of stuff middle America laps up every afternoon at four, delivered by Phil, Oprah and the like.

My mother Rhoda, New England trooper that she is, weathered these appearances with much aplomb. But there was an awkwardness. There was one time in Boston when we had a fight right before the show. Not a big one. I had stayed in bed a little long watching stupid morning TV, enjoying room service. By the time I had finished eating, my mother was already dressed and ready. I leisurely showered. Once in the taxi, I found I'd forgotten the exact address of the studio. The taxi driver was pissed off and drove fast and erratically, even for Boston. There was an enormous amount of traffic. My mother white-knuckled the curves. By the time we arrived at the studio — late — we were hardly speaking. I heard her voice in my head: "If you had gotton out of bed when you were supposed to . . ."

We sat side by side in front of the make-up mirror getting new faces for the bright lights. Rhoda's lips were pursed, the thin line revealing her annoyance. I remember thinking, *I wonder if we'll pull this one off.*

We did, of course, presenting a warm and caring mother/daughter duo even while harboring resentments. Afterwards we ate lunch with a mother/daughter team from the book. I cornered the daughter in the rest room.

"Is it really that good between you two?" I asked the thirty-something lawyer busy scrubbing off her mascara. During the thirty-minute talk show, her mother had acted like her best friend. It seemed the darling daughter's lesbianism had been no more traumatic than a surprise case of the hiccoughs.

"Ha!" she snorted, slipping off the pantyhose and skirt she had donned for the occasion. "We have stuff a mile deep; it's just not about my being gay," she said, slipping on her jeans. "You want to see us fight? Just bring up the subject of my new lover, or my 'insistence' on working as a public defender. Or let's talk about my dad . . . Or the death penalty!"

Things were still not hunky-dory with Rhoda and me. Yes, I

had successfully squelched the anti-lesbian sentiment, though over the years it has reared its dreary head a number of times. I was hugely resentful of my brother's elaborate wedding. She didn't really understand why. And, yes, I am tired of defending the love affair between lesbians and therapy. But these days, Rhoda clips magazine articles about anything gay and has "come out" about me to almost everyone in her life. Surprising to her though not to me, most of the people she told also had something to tell; many revealed a gay or lesbian son, daughter, family member, or friend.

But some "stuff" between us remained despite efforts on both our parts to resolve the queer issue. And over the years I've come to identify it as "old" stuff: sibling rivalry, residual emotions between her, me and my deceased father, resentments stemming from childhood. And then there are things that we just don't like about each other, the kinds of things that only became clear when the brouhaha about lesbiana began to blow over. I am always late — or just barely on time. She wants always to be on time — or early. How do we travel together? With difficulty and compromise.

We started to see our relationship for what it is, what it has been, what it could be, aside from but including my being a lesbian. And this hasn't always been easy. We've had fights and silent standoffs and three-hour long-distance phone calls. We've written long angry letters and short notes of apology. We've also written letters full of respect and love. I am fortunate to have a mother so willing to listen, to do work with me, to put energy into our relationship.

Since publication of *Different Daughters*, I have been giving coming out workshops to college students and community groups, to groups of mothers, daughters and both together. I showed a video featuring mothers from the book talking about their various roads to understanding. On this tape are women who admit their fears, their disappointments. One woman cries and pleads with the mostly-lesbian audience for help in understanding what *happened* to her daughter. Lesbians — and mothers — love the tape. And through watching these relationships — including my own — change, lurch, deepen, and hit potholes, I came to understand that lesbianism is not always the big chasm in family relationships, but often a catalyst for shaking up relationships that were already quite rocky or unresolved.

141

Though careful not to minimize anyone's homophobia, I began to view lesbianism as a handy scapegoat for unresolved anger and resentment, as well as old-fashioned parental disappointment. "Why couldn't my daughter be a lawyer? Now that she's come out she wants to be a social worker."

Once, at the Parents and Friends of Lesbians and Gays national conference in Chicago, I actually heard one mother complain about lesbian potlucks. "What is it about lesbians and potlucks?" she asked, her face quite full of pain. She was dressed immaculately, pearls and a gray cashmere suit. "Why can't she give a dinner party like everyone else?" I assured her there were lesbians who gave dinner parties, and straight people who held potlucks, but I don't think I fully convinced her. I saw her at the break, bending the sympathetic ear of another finely dressed woman. Their conversation was about *futons*. "Yes! They sleep right on the floor!" the other exclaimed. The problem was obvious to me: This woman's attachment to her class was fueling her resentment of her daughter's "lifestyle." "*Everyone* in Japan sleeps on the floor," I quipped as I walked past them.

But mothers were not the only ones to blame sexuality for all their daughters' foibles. (Not that a futon on the floor is a foible — don't get me wrong!) One recently-out lesbian complained that her parents were unsupportive of her female lover. I asked, "Were they supportive of the men you dated before you came out?" "Hmm . . ." she said. "Not really."

Take the oft-heard: "My mother hates what I wear." Really, ladies, isn't this a given? Can we really pin this on queerness? Even my straight friends say their mothers don't approve of how they dress. As both sides complained, I tried to unravel the threads. Mothers: Did you ever approve of your daughters' choices? Sure, you might not like her hair style, but do you have the right to dictate a twenty-year-old's grooming habits? Aren't schisms common to all mother/daughter relationships? The queer quotient is often used to justify already entrenched family dynamics.

None of this is easy. Not for me and not for the rest of us trying to sort out family relationships and our place in the world. Often it's easier to blame everything on homophobia than to dive into deeper waters. Better to dig in your heels at the edge of the pit than fall head first into the muck. Who wants to sort through that old stuff, especially with your parents?

In hindsight I can see that *Different Daughters* was crucial to my journey towards family acceptance. It was simple: I wanted my mother to like me and I started by addressing what I thought was the most serious obstacle to that goal. But now I see my lesbianism more as a part of my life, part of the package of who I am, sometimes why my mother and I get along, and sometimes why we don't.

The letters I receive from mothers are usually from those in the first stages of this work. They are relieved to read a book about women like themselves telling the truth about their feelings. We all need that. Sadly enough, most of them have no one to talk to, and they are often isolated from their own family members. For the most part they are alone, dealing bravely with their own misunderstandings and guilt. Every letter I receive strikes me as a blessing; somewhere there's a lesbian whose mother cares enough about her to start this work.

Different Daughters has brought comfort and community to many women, both mothers and daughters, and I am thrilled to have helped those stories of love and pain and confusion come to light. But if things aren't peachy in your family of origin, even after you've explained the politics of lesbian separatism and — gasp — what we do in bed, I'm not surprised. There's more, and it's not all connected to lavender and labryses.

Rhoda and I are still working on our relationship, a process which will continue forever, I suspect. This work is about acceptance, but not only of my sexual preference: acceptance of her by me, me by her.

But there are still times she doesn't like my haircuts — and vice versa. Right before my last visit home, I made the mistake of telling my mom I had just had my hair cut.

"Short?" she asked, her voice betraying her disapproval.

"No, Mom," I said. "I had it cut long."

DYKES AND FAGS:
WHAT'S GOING DOWN?

Michigan," I said again. "Does it mean anything to you?"
My friend Tommy looked at me blankly. He swiveled in the restaurant booth to query his partner. Mark shrugged.

"Every lesbian knows what 'Michigan' means," I told them. "Are you sure you don't have any idea?"

"Something about the lakes?" Tom ventured. "The water? Wetness?"

I asked our waiter, a strutting gay blade.

"No," he said. "Nothing," he set down coffee, fingered his string of pearls. "Zip."

Over dessert I explained the Michigan Womyn's Music Festival to Tommy and Mark. For a week every August in upstate Michigan, thousands of lesbians gather from all over the globe. Michigan is a plot of "womyn's land," sometimes hot and dry, sometimes cold and wet, where dykes come to pitch tents and commune with each other and nature. Michigan means naked nymphs and a return to what many lesbians refer to as "home."

Mark slid his Armani specs low on his nose. Tommy rolled his baby-blue eyes, "You're kidding!"

I assured them (while enjoying the last bite of Tommy's double-fudge pie) that Michigan was not something I could make up.

Then I elaborated, detailing my one and only experience as a "festy-goer." Five years ago, in my late twenties, curious and game for anything, I hit Michigan in the middle of a Midwest book tour, my best friend in tow. It was the year of constant downpour, and I remember waking up from a vaguely erotic dream to find that the wetness I felt was due to the four inches of water pooling in my tent.

"I saw more bared breasts than I ever wanted to," I told Tommy.

"And fought continuously with the lesbo-rangers about where I had chosen to pitch camp. Every morning I received a note from them citing my 'inappropriate' camping spot and stating that I would have to move. Having sought out my secluded site for privacy, I had yet to see any reason to move so I refused to unearth my soggy tent. Finally one night after a concert I wandered back to my tent only to find that I had actually camped right next to the scheduled midnight S/M workshop."

Tommy laughed. "Did you attend?" he asked, raising an eye brow. "Do tell."

"I stayed long enough to see this poor women who was tied to a tree get stung by some insect and start crying."

I continued my Michigan spiel. I told about the crunchy-tofu-vego-lacto food. Piles of nondescript rabbit food prepared by volunteers in vats big enough to cook a rhino. "I spent most of my time at the coffee and donuts stand trying to stay dry."

"No men, *anywhere*?" Tommy queried.

"The only men who come 'on the land' are there to empty the 'Porta-Janes.' And as they come on, there's a relay of women preceding them, chanting a chorus of 'Men on the land! Men on the land!'"

Tommy ran his fingers through his curly, graying hair. "I can't believe it!" He scanned the table for the last of his pie. I flashed a guilty smile and signaled the waiter for another. All three of us are in our mid-thirties, watching our waistlines, but hey . . .

I told more. About the throngs of lesbo groupies, fighting for a fling with a "star." About the political in-fighting that always takes center stage despite top caliber music from internationally known out and not-so-out women performers. "There are always women who want to shut down the S/Mers," I explained. "And *dyke-cotts* — lesbian versions of boycotts."

Tommy hooted. "Enough, enough!"

Tom and Mark went home and questioned their friends, several "kinds" of gay men, especially targeting the ones who hang with girls. Not one of them had ever heard of Michigan. A camp-out with ten thousand dykes? "Oh my god," one said, genuinely a little frightened. "The things I don't know . . ."

Tom and Mark are genuine dyke spikes. What else do you call fags who hang with lesbians? I met them at their home several years ago. They moved in across from my best friends in a neighborhood we now refer to as "Homo Heights." We all live in Provincetown, here on the tip of Cape Cod, the left arm extending eastward into the Atlantic from the state of Massachusetts.

Provincetown is a place where gay men and lesbians genuinely mix. For several decades it has been a gay vacation mecca, a haven for artists and writers. Now a number of communities make it home year round. And — what? — maybe a little less than half of us resident P-towners are gay. Overall there's a rough weaving of traditional straight families, working class mostly, the Portuguese fishing community, the alternative artists/writers scene, and the various gay and lesbian clans. And here too is diversity: leather queens, boy businessmen, political dyke separatists, lipstick lesbians, and well-known gay and lesbian performers who make this their off-touring home.

In the winter the population scatters, dwindles, or flies south, and only a few thousand of us of any kind are left clinging to the tip of this sandy spit. In the summer when throngs of both straight and gay tourists descend, the population multiplies to upwards of fifty thousand.

Thus our unique town breeds a special kind of interdependence among gays and lesbians. We work together and play together. In the summer we kick up our heels at the same dance bars, frequent the same beach — although for the most part we position ourselves at opposite ends.

On warm nights we sit together on the curb in front of the one late-night café ogling and gossiping until well past midnight. This café, Spiritus, is Provincetown's drive-in *sans* carhops. It's a tiny café by city standards, serving high-priced coffee and somewhat soggy pizza. The aroma of Spiritus extends well past the twenty feet of patio which fronts the main street. The smells of coffee and pizza blend with the classic fugitive bar smells: cigarette smoke clinging to sweat-soaked, sunburned bodies. In the off-season, when the front of Spiritus is boarded up and crested with snow, we P-towners meet elsewhere for more coffee and at the myriad arty/literati events.

So you would think we gays and lesbians live similar lives. You might even think we know much about each other's lives.

And for the most part you'd be wrong.

I don't even know what amyl nitrate smells like.

"Like old socks with an acid chaser," Tommy has told me.

"Hmmm," I say, not for a moment understanding the appeal.

Mark and Tommy don't exclusively hang with women, in fact they're intimately connected to many groups in this small gay village. They are refugees from the big city; they came here to live a quieter life, to move at a slower pace. Mark traded his fast-paced NYC job for one here in Provincetown — one of about three in the whole place — but he still makes it home for lunch every day. (Tommy cooked him "white trash" yesterday: reheated spaghetti over cottage cheese with a hot dog side. He'll kill me for telling.) While Mark is out slaving over a warm computer, Tommy works in the basement, sculpting. We call them "the boys" and our lives connect over "Star Trek," rented movies (fodder against the long, boring winter) and town gossip.

Why do they hang with women? I don't know for sure. Tommy really likes women — a rare quality in a gay man. In fact, in his early twenties he was married — twice. And why do we girls hang with them when we live in the midst of lesbo heaven? Shared interests, curiosity, diversity. Sometimes it's less intense to fraternize with fellows. We like 'em. They're funny. And it seems that in the overall scope of gay/lesbian relations, which historically have never been that smooth, it's time to finally get friendly with each other.

And besides, Tommy has been my guide to the nether world of gay culture. Culture? What does it mean that the guys know exactly who in town is biggest? (And I'm not talking tallest.) He tells gay gossip of the Hollywood variety; which dead artist left his sex-toy collection in a suitcase that was auctioned off as old luggage. He tells about the proclivities of various knowns and unknowns.

"No!" we gasp. It's like we're in third grade: "The boys do *what*?"

Us girls might do the same things, but we do them so differently. Take for instance cruising. Beach cruising. Women make surreptitious eye contact, catch an eye, try to make sense of the pattern of beach blankets surrounding our object of fancy. Is that a lover she's sharing that towel with? Her ex-lover? Does it mean anything that she's massaging oil into her back? No, there's more than six inches between them. Okay, what's she reading . . .

Meanwhile the guys are already off doing it in the dunes.

And at Spiritus. We women hang out in gangs of three or four. We watch other gals in groups stroll the promenade, duck into the bar across the street. Maybe there is a glance over a shoulder, later a look across a crowd. Perhaps even a dance, and on a rare and lucky occasion, a *date* . . . Girls usually meet girls through friends (and at those proverbial lesbian potlucks — it's true!). This makes us oh-so-poor at cruising.

The guys? They spot a hunk and then — with a look, a small gesture — they're off to the beach, or to the "boatyard," the infamous lover's lane of P-town fairy folk tales.

A lot of our "differences" do gather under the loose awning of sex. I mean, I've been as out there as the best of them, but I've never gone to a party where I had to check my clothes.

("Yes," Tommy assures. "You hang your clothes in a room — which is usually locked — and then you get them in the morning at check out."

"What if you want to leave?"

"You don't.")

And I was a bit shocked when Tommy called to say that the enema machine (what?) was being transported from across the street (a notorious sex-party house) for a big bash somewhere down the road. He swears it's true.

But I, too, can make Tommy blush. "*Strap on*," I say in a discussion about women's sex toys. He flushes neck upwards. Talk of what size a dyke's dildo should be — your own or your gal-pal's, or should you own an array?) — left him stuttering.

"My virgin ears," he said and camped a grimace.

And although he himself knows better, he reported on a friend who was flabbergasted to learn that women had — really! — *three* holes!

I walked into the café the other day with a copy of *Blueboy* under my arm. For those of you out-of-the-know, *Blueboy* is a fag rag on the nice end of the spectrum (opposite *Manmeat*.) There are glossy naked boys, trim and blonde, alongside travel articles and smatterings of gay news and politics. Apparently this is most radical: *Blueboy* is billed as the "thinking man's" magazine. Yikes.

The guys in the café were appalled — where did I get it? What was I doing with it? Most importantly, did I know that the guy on the cover worked at the local health food store last summer and went out with . . . ?

As lesbians follow in the . . . *er* . . . footsteps of our gay brothers perhaps our differences won't look so extreme. The current "sex-positive" hoopla finds lesbians talking about sex more often. Maybe women are even *having* more sex. If my gang is any indicator, we've come a long way — so to speak — towards bringing our sexuality out of the closet. We've got lesbo sex magazines and even sex clubs, and now "hot" refers to more than the weather. I don't know where all this is leading us women, but I doubt we'll be having anonymous sex at rest stops like some of our male counterparts. I may be wrong; I've been wrong before.

Tommy says I'm wrong. "Dead wrong," he says, and we both feel the chill.

Tommy thinks lesbians are well on their way to copying the sexual behavior of gay men in the seventies and eighties.

"How much will you girls learn from having watched us live through it?" he asks, putting strange emphasis on the word live. He knows many of us don't practice safe sex. Will lesbians tread the path of multiple partners, open relationships, fuck-buddies? And then circle back to monogamy and marriage?

We talk endlessly about this stuff. He's been up, down, around and through the gay male sex scene, from deep in the Village in NYC to this little drip of sand out here off the coast of New England. He's tried about every which way to do it and has ended up settled and coupled, sometimes uneasily so, but content with his choice. He and Mark tend their unbelievably beautiful garden, babying bulbs and clipping roses and arguing over the placement of the myriad annuals. They walk their dog on the beach, **live** a domestic life. And I'm single, watching from the outside, not knowing exactly in which direction I will turn. Towards marriage or fuck-buddies? Something in between?

Meanwhile, sandwiched in the folds of *Blueboy*, the feature article on sex covered spirituality, relationships, therapy, even — gasp — intimacy. Sound familiar girls? Tommy tells me that boys are learning to *process*. That they are starting to talk about feelings and *intimacy*. This is something we know how to do *ad nauseam*. Evidence: Now all the girls and about *half* the guys in town are going to therapy. It seems the boys are also riding *our* wake.

Dykes and fags don't really know much about one another, but cross-pollination is occurring. Sure, many women came up and out through the feminist fracas and distrusted and shunned the entire male gender for a good many years. But now we've been living together for a while, especially in such places as Provincetown. And — surprise — we all like each other.

What will we learn? Will gay men, who seem to be finding voice and power in political organizing, seek advice from lesbians? Can we offer each other our experiences, each from his or her corner?

I, for one, have a ton to say about endless meetings and — ouch — *consensus*. (Like don't even attempt it!)

Kidding aside, through political work women have learned to listen to each other, and most importantly acknowledge privileges of skin color, education, social and class status. Much of what we've learned has come through bitter fighting and with much pain. Now I see men trying to build coalitions and challenge the world without doing the deeper work of challenging themselves, acknowledging their own privilege. Watch out.

All this is part of a larger discussion, a historical overview that will no doubt be tackled by some young queer in academia. In the meantime, both here in Provincetown and elsewhere, we dykes and fags are getting to know each other. On a recent spring afternoon I sat outside in Tommy's garden. The crocuses were just popping through, points of yellow and purple which stung the gray earth. While rooting around, strangling stray weeds, Tommy took the opportunity to ask me some more anthropological questions.

"And those hatchet things around their necks?"

I explain about the battle-axes swinging from the throats of half our summer visitors. "No, they're not some sort of implement for cleaning fingernails. They represent the double-edged axes of our Amazon foremothers."

He rolls his eyes. I can tell that sometimes he find us so, well, *kitsch* . . .

"You'll love the idea of Contact Dykes," I say and laugh, because I know he'll think this is really kitsch.

"*Contact* Dykes?" he asks. "What can that possibly . . ."

I tell him about *Lesbian Connection*, a grass roots publication that spans the hinterlands of this country. Yes, *Lesbian Connection* runs a listing of gals — said Contact Dykes — hither and thither who welcome calls, inquires, even guests if you're of the tribe. "So, if you're visiting Omaha you can just take out your *L.C.* and look one up," I explain.

"Like a 'find the lesbians' hand-out?" Tommy asks, somewhat sarcastically.

"Okay, okay, we girls *do* need help finding each other. We can't just pull up to the public park and watch who strolls by."

Our info exchange is ongoing. Me? I picture myself as Margaret Mead, notebook in hand and consistently amazed.

"So when exactly is the festival?" Tommy's kneeling next to a rose bush. He looks great in a dress and is dying to sneak into Michigan.

Books from Cleis Press

Fiction

Another Love by Erzsébet Galgóczi. ISBN: 0-939416-52-2 24.95 cloth;
ISBN: 0-939416-51-4 8.95 paper.

Cosmopolis: Urban Stories by Women edited by Ines Rieder. ISBN: 0-939416-36-0
24.95 cloth; ISBN: 0-939416-37-9 9.95 paper.

Night Train To Mother by Ronit Lentin. ISBN: 0-939416-29-8 24.95 cloth;
ISBN: 0-939416-28-X 9.95 paper.

The One You Call Sister: New Women's Fiction edited by Paula Martinac.
ISBN: 0-939416-30-1 24.95 cloth; ISBN: 0-939416031-X 9.95 paper.

Queer and Pleasant Danger: Writing Out My Life by Louise Rafkin.
ISBN: 0-939416-60-3 24.95 cloth; ISBN: 0-939416-61-1 9.95 paper.

Unholy Alliances: New Women's Fiction edited by Louise Rafkin.
ISBN: 0-939416-14-X 21.95 cloth; ISBN: 0-939416-15-8 9.95 paper.

The Wall by Marlen Haushofer. ISBN: 0-939416-53-0 24.95 cloth;
ISBN: 0-939416-54-9 paper.

Sexuality/Lesbian Studies

A Lesbian Love Advisor by Celeste West. ISBN: 0-939416-27-1 24.95 cloth;
ISBN: 0-939416-26-3 9.95 paper.

Boomer: Railroad Memoirs by Linda Niemann. ISBN: 0-939416-55-7 12.95 paper.

Different Daughters: A Book by Mothers of Lesbians edited by Louise Rafkin.
ISBN: 0-939416-12-3 21.95 cloth; ISBN: 0-939416-13-1 9.95 paper.

Different Mothers: Sons & Daughters of Lesbians Talk About Their Lives edited by
Louise Rafkin. ISBN: 0-939416-40-9 24.95 cloth; ISBN: 0-939416-41-7
9.95 paper.

Good Sex: Real Stories From Real People by Julia Hutton. ISBN: 0-939416-56-5
24.95 cloth; ISBN: 0-939416-57-3 12.95 paper.

Long Way Home: The Odyssey of a Lesbian Mother and Her Children by Jeanne Jullion.
ISBN: 0-939416-05-0 8.95 paper.

More Serious Pleasure: Lesbian Erotic Stories and Poetry edited by the Sheba Collective.
ISBN: 0-939416-48-4 24.95 cloth; ISBN: 0-939416-47-6 9.95 paper.

The Night Audrey's Vibrator Spoke: A Stonewall Riots Collection by Andrea Natalie.
ISBN: 0-939416-64-6 8.95 paper.

Serious Pleasure: Lesbian Erotic Stories and Poetry edited by the Sheba Collective.
ISBN: 0-939416-46-8 24.95 cloth; ISBN: 0-939416-45-X 9.95 paper.

Sex Work: Writings by Women in the Sex Industry edited by Frédérique Delacoste
and Priscilla Alexander. ISBN: 0-939416-10-7 24.95 cloth;
ISBN: 0-939416-11-5 16.95 paper.

Susie Bright's Sexual Reality: A Virtual Sex World Reader. ISBN: 0-939416-58-1 24.95 cloth; ISBN: 0-939416-59-X 9.95 paper

Susie Sexpert's Lesbian Sex World by Susie Bright. ISBN: 0-939416-34-4 24.95 cloth; ISBN: 0-939416-35-2 9.95 paper.

Women's Studies

Peggy Deery: An Irish Family at War by Nell McCafferty. ISBN: 0-939416-38-7 24.95 cloth; ISBN: 0-939416-39-5 9.95 paper.

The Shape of Red: Insider/Outsider Reflections by Ruth Hubbard and Margaret Randall. ISBN: 0-939416-19-0 24.95 cloth; ISBN: 0-939416-18-2 9.95 paper.

Women & Honor: Some Notes on Lying by Adrienne Rich. ISBN: 0-939416-44-1 3.95 paper.

Latin American Studies

Beyond the Border: A New Age in Latin American Women's Fiction edited by Nora Erro-Peralta and Caridad Silva-Núñez. ISBN: 0-939416-42-5 24.95 cloth; ISBN: 0-939416-43-3 12.95 paper.

The Little School: Tales of Disappearance and Survival in Argentina by Alicia Partnoy. ISBN: 0-939416-08-5 21.95 cloth; ISBN: 0-939416-07-7 9.95 paper.

You Can't Drown the Fire: Latin American Women Writing in Exile edited by Alicia Partnoy. ISBN: 0-939416-16-6 24.95 cloth; ISBN: 0-939416-17-4 9.95 paper.

Health/Recovery Titles:

The Absence of the Dead Is Their Way of Appearing by Mary Winfrey Trautmann. ISBN: 0-939416-04-2 8.95 paper.

AIDS: The Women edited by Ines Rieder and Patricia Ruppelt. ISBN: 0-939416-20-4 24.95 cloth; ISBN: 0-939416-21-2 9.95 paper

Don't: A Woman's Word by Elly Danica. ISBN: 0-939416-23-9 21.95 cloth; ISBN: 0-939416-22-0 8.95 paper

1 in 3: Women with Cancer Confront an Epidemic edited by Judith Brady. ISBN: 0-939416-50-6 24.95 cloth; ISBN: 0-939416-49-2 10.95 paper.

Voices in the Night: Women Speaking About Incest edited by Toni A.H. McNaron and Yarrow Morgan. ISBN: 0-939416-02-6 9.95 paper.

With the Power of Each Breath: A Disabled Women's Anthology edited by Susan Browne, Debra Connors and Nanci Stern. ISBN: 0-939416-09-3 24.95 cloth; ISBN: 0-939416-06-9 10.95 paper.

Woman-Centered Pregnancy and Birth by the Federation of Feminist Women's Health Centers. ISBN: 0-939416-03-4 11.95 paper.

Animal Rights

And a Deer's Ear, Eagle's Song and Bear's Grace: Relationships Between Animals and Women edited by Theresa Corrigan and Stephanie T. Hoppe.
ISBN: 0-939416-38-7 24.95 cloth; ISBN: 0-939416-39-5 9.95 paper.

With a Fly's Eye, Whale's Wit and Woman's Heart: Relationships Between Animals and Women edited by Theresa Corrigan and Stephanie T. Hoppe.
ISBN: 0-939416-24-7 24.95 cloth; ISBN: 0-939416-25-5 9.95 paper.

Since 1980, Cleis Press has published progressive books by women. We welcome your order and will ship your books as quickly as possible. Individual orders must be prepaid (U.S. dollars only). Please add 15% shipping. PA residents add 6% sales tax. Mail orders: Cleis Press, PO Box 8933, Pittsburgh PA 15221. MasterCard and Visa orders: $25 minimum—include account number, exp. date, and signature. FAX your credit card order: (412) 937-1567. Or, phone us Mon-Fri, 9 am - 5 pm EST: (412) 937-1555.